The Incredible 5-Point Scale:
The Significantly Improved and Expanded Second Edition

*Assisting students in understanding social interactions
and controlling their emotional responses*

Kari Dunn Buron and Mitzi Curtis
2 teachers from Minnesota

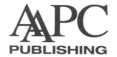
PUBLISHING

P.O. Box 23173
Shawnee Mission, Kansas 66283-0173
www.aapcpublishing.net

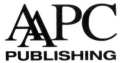

©2012 AAPC Publishing
P.O. Box 23173
Shawnee Mission, Kansas 66283-0173
www.aapcpublishing.net

Publisher's Cataloging-in-Publication

Buron, Kari Dunn.

    The incredible 5-point scale / assisting students in understanding social interactions and controlling their emotional responses / Kari Dunn Buron and Mitzi Curtis. -- Significantly improved and expanded 2nd ed. -- Shawnee Mission, Kan. : AAPC Publishing, c2012.

    ISBN: 978-1-937473-07-5
    LCCN: 2012942651
    At head of title: Evidence-based practice.
    Updated and expanded edtion of the 2003 book.
    Includes bibliographical references.
    Blank scales, small portable scales, and scale worksheets are downloadable from www.aapcpublishing.net/9936 for easy duplication.

    1. Autistic children--Behavior modification. 2. Children with autism spectrum disorders--Behavior modification--Study and teaching. 3. Autistic children--Life skills guides. 4. Social skills in children--Study and teaching. 5. Social interaction in children--Study and teaching. 6. Interpersonal relations in children--Study and teaching. 7. Autistic children--Education. 8. Children with autism spectrum disorders--Education. 9. Teachers of children with disabilities--Handbooks, manuals, etc. I. Curtis, Mitzi. II. Title. III. Title: Incredible five-point scale.

RJ506.A9 B87 2012
618.92/85882--dc23   1208

This book is designed in Elven and Century Schoolbook.

Printed in the United States of America.

This book is dedicated to
systemized thinkers everywhere ...
we have written this for you.

Contents

Preface

In this second edition of the bestselling *The Incredible 5-Point Scale* (Buron & Curtis, 2003), we have divided the book into six sections. The first section is a brief overview of how to use the 5-Point Scale, along with some stories about its use that we have gathered over the years. The second section includes the specifics of our original 14 scales and scenarios as a reminder for readers of the first book and as a background and introduction for newcomers to this incredible tool. The remainder of the book presents brand-new material, prompted by demands of practitioners across the country and abroad for scales that are applicable to younger students and those on the more severe end of the autism spectrum. Thus, the third section introduces scales specifically designed for younger children, whereas the fourth section addresses individuals with more classic forms of autism, including an expanded use of the Anxiety Curve model. The fifth section includes a variety of new scale ideas we have used successfully since the original book was printed. Finally, the sixth section is a list of goals and objectives related to the use of the scale that teachers have used on individualized education programs (IEPs). Blank scales, small portable scales, and scale worksheets are downloadable at http://www.aapcpublishing.net/9936 for easy duplication.

Some Background Information

We introduced *The Incredible 5-Point Scale* in 2003 as a method of teaching social understanding to students with autism spectrum disorders (ASD) and similar challenges. Since that time, we have learned more about why the scale works and how to use scales effectively with diverse populations.

Despite the recent emergence of some exciting new social curricula, the idea of teaching social competence is just beginning to gain attention in teacher preparation programs. What we have learned in the past nine years is that individuals on the spectrum need to be directly taught information we had previously thought of as "common knowledge." To paraphrase Daniel Goleman in *The Brain and Emotional Intelligence: New Insights* (2011), the range of what we think and do is limited to what we fail to notice ... Individuals with ASD seem to fail to notice that they are failing to notice, and this failure to notice shapes their thoughts and behaviors. A primary goal of the scale is to help them notice and functionally respond to their own and others' social behavior.

The objective of the 5-Point Scale is to teach social and emotional information in a concrete, systematic, and non-judging way. Students who have poor skills in the areas of social thinking or emotional regulation often exhibit challenging behaviors, particularly when facing difficult social situations. In the scale, teachers and parents have a simple, yet effective way to teach social rules and expectations and, along with the individual with ASD, problem-solve behavioral responses of others, troubleshoot past and future social scenarios, and create plans for self-management.

Simon Baron-Cohen's empathizing-systemizing theory (Golan & Baron-Cohen, 2008) seems to support the idea of using a scale to teach social and emotional concepts. The theory suggests that individuals on the autism spectrum have a strong desire to analyze information to determine what causes what, and implies that by using a system to teach difficult information, we are making use of the person's learning strengths.

Using the 5-Point Scale is a great way for all caregivers to communicate more effectively. Once a scale is developed for voice volume, frustration level, or any other issue, situations faced at home and at school can be plugged into the system so that everyone begins to speak the same language. For example, if a voice-level scale is developed at school, parents can use the same defined voice levels to communicate with their child at home. A #4 might be an outside voice, whether it is at home or at school. A #2 voice may be a library voice at school, but can also be a voice to use at home when the baby is napping. Grandma and Grandpa can then post the scale in their home to communicate when and where different voice volumes should be used.

Individuals who exhibit challenging behaviors are most likely lacking the skills needed to negotiate social interactions effectively. That is, if they find themselves failing over and over again at social interactions, the issue inevitably gets personal. Thus, it is likely that a person who is not very good at something that everyone else seems to do seamlessly will develop some pretty defensive feelings about the issue. For this reason, it is important to keep "judging words" out of the scales. For example, avoid the use of "good" and "bad" or "right" and "wrong." Also keep out frustrating words like "consequences" or "inappropriate."

If you are addressing issues that are against the law, your scale might look like this:

Rules*

Rating	What This Looks Like
5	These behaviors are against the law, like hitting or destroying property. Even if you don't agree with them, they are still against the law.
4	These behaviors might be scary but not illegal, like swearing at someone or using other mean words. These behaviors can get you fired from a job or cause other people to avoid you.
3	These behaviors might create problems at school, at work, or at home, but they are not scary. Examples include standing too close to someone, talking too loudly, and forgetting to share.
2	These behaviors might not create big problems. They might include things like ignoring other people. These behaviors probably won't get you into trouble, but they are usually not helpful if you are trying to create friendships and relationships.
1	These behaviors might actually help cause other people to feel good about you. These are relationship actions.

In the above example, issues are dealt with in a very direct and honest way, but typical judging words are avoided. Simply put, just address the facts and be *compassionately*

---

* This is similar to what Temple Grandin calls "social sins" (http://www.iidc.indiana.edu/index.php?pageId=600).

honest. Here is another example of addressing an issue directly but without judgment:

Meeting Girls

Rating	What This Looks Like	What Is the Girl Likely to Think?
5	Telling a girl she has a good body	This is not really welcomed by most girls. It might sound creepy if the girl doesn't know you well and might even seem aggressive.
4	Singing a song to a girl across a crowded room	Even though this is not harmful, it might seem strange, and the girl might end up feeling embarrassed.
3	Fluttering your eye lashes at a girl	This is confusing. The girl will probably not know what to think.
2	Joining a club or theater group after school specifically to meet girls	This is OK, but remember that you might not meet a girl you like or who likes you. Be patient
1	Sitting next to a girl in class and introducing yourself	This is good. Keep it simple.

Another good way to increase a person's acceptance of a scale, and motivation to use the scale, is to *co-create* the scale. We have found that this can even be done with very young children and children who have very limited verbal skills. One way to get input from individuals who are unable or reluctant to speak is to use the activity called *A 5 Could Make Me Lose Control* (Buron, 2007). This activity allows the person to problem-solve nonverbally by placing word or picture cards of various environments or social situations, such as Getting Into an Argument, into pockets listed 1-5. The situations placed in pocket #1 do not bother her at all; situations in pocket #2 might make her feel uneasy; situations in pocket #3 might make her feel nervous; situations in pocket #4 might make her angry; and, finally, situations in pocket #5 might make her lose control or even explode.

Co-created scales for a person who is higher functioning might take the form of a worksheet. This gives the person the opportunity to fill in how specific things might make him feel and strategies he will use to control those feelings. Such co-created scales can be used to design support plans by adding support to the environments that seem to cause problems.

Some teachers and parents have asked us if the scale needs to include five levels. Although there is nothing magical about the number 5, it does seem to be the easiest number to use. Trying to break every social concept or emotion into 10 parts, for example, seems too hard. Nevertheless, we have encountered many students who have created their own scales, and a few of them have insisted on including 3, 7, 8, and 10 points. We even met a young man who created a 15-point scale.

Keep in mind that the idea is to help the person understand social and emotional concepts by breaking the concept into parts. If he grasps the system and wants to add levels, this might be a sign that he is not only embracing the system but enjoying the activity by playing with it. If that is the case, by all means, support him. We want him to embrace the system, so you don't want to hinder that goal by insisting on the number 5. We are trying to teach social flexibility after all.

Perhaps at its best, the scale can teach self-management skills. In the book *When My Worries Get Too Big!* (Buron, 2006), the scale is used to teach young children to recognize when their bodies are stressed and to give them ideas for managing their emotions. The original "check-in" scale has been expanded over the years, and we have found that it can be used effectively to teach emotional regulation. Students who exhibit high levels of anxiety can begin to "check in" on a regular basis throughout the day to stay on top of big emotions. If they find that they are experiencing even a little stress, then relaxation routines can be implemented to avoid a loss of control.

Sample Check-in Scale

Rating	How It Feels and What I Can Do
5	**OUT OF CONTROL!** I need to spend time in a safe place to calm my nerves. Listen to Adele on headphones.
4	**Very upset or angry.** I will stay in the resource room for a while and work through my nervous feelings with Mrs. Wilson.
3	**Not very good.** I am not feeling well today. I did not get much sleep or maybe I had a bad bus ride. I need to do some relaxation exercises to help.
2	**OK.** I can go back to class and continue my day. I can practice my positive self-talk to keep me calm.
1	**Good day.** I am having a good day. I feel calm and focused. Good to go to class. ☺

Daniel Goleman (2011) explains emotional intelligence as the interplay between self-awareness, social awareness, self-management, and relationship management. In this edition of *The Incredible 5-Point Scale*, we offer examples of how the scale has been used to address each of these four cognitive areas.

In closing, thank you to everyone who used the scale and took the time to let us know. Your stories have been inspiring, and we hope they are reflected in this edition.

Enjoy!

Kari and Mitzi

Introduction

Using the Scale

It is important to remember that a scale is a teaching tool. It is not simply another behavior management strategy. Nor is it a miracle that you can just post on the wall and hope things will change.

We recommend following these steps when creating a scale, preferably working together with the person for whom the scale is designed:

1. Determine the problem. What is the person doing that you wish he wasn't? Or what is he not doing that you wish he was? What is the social situation he seems to be confused by?
2. Identify the skill or social concept the person needs to be taught in order to do this better.
3. Break that concept into five parts. Make #1 the smallest and #5 the biggest (avoid the terms "good" and "bad").
4. Use a story or a simple memo, even a video, to help the person understand what the scale is all about and how to use it.
5. Review the scale with the person prior to predictably difficult times or when he has to be in predictably difficult environments.
6. Use the scale in real situations by prompting the person using a small portable scale.
7. Create a portable scale for the person to carry as a reminder.

Here are some examples of concepts or situations where a scale has been used to successfully teach individuals ranging in age and severity of challenges:

- personal distance
- voice volume
- what is fair
- tone of voice
- speed in the hallway
- fear
- worrying
- asking for help
- emotions
- distractions
- who is a friend

- sexual behavior
- self-advocacy
- energy level
- friendships
- losing and winning
- what is funny
- perspective taking
- is it a problem?
- competition
- problems
- touching

- tolerance for others
- anger
- how other people think
- words we use
- changes
- breaking the law
- classroom rules
- bus rides
- sadness
- manners
- looking at other people

While self-regulation is not addressed in the common core standards, it is an essential skill. Students with self-regulation skills are ready to learn information addressed in the standards. Children and adolescents with regulation challenges are not ready to learn. They and their teachers spend time addressing the behaviors resulting from self-regulation problems. The Incredible 5-Point Scale, a visual self-management support, helps individuals learn self-regulation skills so that they are ready to learn the skills that will lead to school and life success.

The Ultimate Goal

A primary goal of the scale is to teach social and emotional information that often eludes persons on the autism spectrum. Initially, the caregiver might need to gather information about the problem and create a scale. This is often the case for very young children or those who are nonverbal. As soon as possible, prompt the person, regardless of age or ability, to interact with the scale. This could include checking in regarding anxiety levels, or simply pointing to a #2 on a voice scale and modeling a whisper voice. This can lead to another goal of the scale, teaching self-management.

Although a story, memo, or video is often used to introduce the use of a scale, after the system has been learned, scales can be developed as a way of "debriefing" after an unexpected problem. Once learned, a scale can even be used "in the moment" to clarify information for the person in a functional, nonthreatening, and nonverbal way.

After one scale has been used successfully, you can use other scales in the same way. For example, once you have made a worries scale, if the person has difficulty with voice volume, you can show her how to use the scale for voice volume. The scale then becomes a predictable system for teaching and learning difficult concepts.

Scale Stories That Make Us Feel Good

Over the past nine years we have had many fun experiences with the scale. Also, others have written to us to share their stories. The following are just a few examples. We hope they make you feel good, too.

We'll start ...

A memorable day for me was when I was providing one-to-one instruction to a fourth-grade boy in math. I was sitting next to him, but that day I was up and down a lot, distracted by knocks at the door and staff asking me questions. The student finally said, "Ms. Curtis, you have way too much energy. You are a 5!" I agreed, and promptly got a therapy ball to sit on.
– Mitzi

I was working at a local elementary school when the morning announcements came on over the loud speaker. The principal began discussing the problem of roughhousing on the bus. The student I was working with looked at me, indicating the voice from the speaker, and said, "That guy is at a 4."
– Kari

Now you ...

I have a great story about a highly verbal four-year-old who knew the scale well. One day when I was in her room, the teacher asked me to help her with a circle activity, and I happened to say, "Well, I will try but it might be hard." Then my student called out, "Don't worry, Mary Beth. It might feel like a 4, but it is only a 2."
— Mary Beth Solheim, a teacher from Minnetonka, Minnesota

When my son was in the ninth grade, we sent him to a Bible camp with limited support. He called home the evening of the fifth day of camp and explained that he had ripped up his scale and thrown it at a counselor. I asked him to tell me what had upset him, but he had little to offer. However, when I asked where he was on his 5-Point Scale, he said "10." I directed him to pack his bag, let the counselor know I was coming, and stay put in his cabin until I got there (he can get a bit aggressive when really agitated or scared). When I arrived, I found out that for the entire time at camp, they had not been in bed before 1:30 a.m., had been out late playing night games and my son had only showered once and brushed his teeth a few times. He had no words to share this with me but was able to communicate through the scale.
— Jody Van Ness, a mom from Minnesota

The 5-Point Scale really helps by being able to say, "I'm at a 2, almost a 3," etc., since I am not always able to communicate how I feel, especially during problem situations. So your scale simply gives me a voice, in a simple form.
— Chloe Rothschild, a 19-year-old from Toledo, Ohio

I was observing a kindergarten class when the teacher stood up in the front of the class and said, "Let's hear Scooby Doo at a 4!" The children yelled, "Scooby Doo!" in loud voices. The teacher then said, "Now let's do Scooby Doo at a 2." The children responded with, "Scooby Doo," using soft voices. The teacher said, "Yes, that's what I need to hear, Scooby Doo at a 2."
— Joyce Santo, a teacher from Roseville, Minnesota

I am a special education teacher who has used the 5-Point Scale for many different things with my students. However, the biggest gift the scale has given me is the ability to help my sister, Amy, who has been suffering with complex posttraumatic stress disorder, dissociative disorder, depersonalization disorder, anxiety, and bipolar disorder. We were able to create a 5-Point Scale that gave her a simple way to let us know what she needed, including rushing her to the hospital once. All of the key people in her life carry her scale, and when she text messages us a number, we know what she is feeling and what she needs us to do. This was the first time we were able to understand what was happening with her. It was the first time we all felt relief because, finally, she wasn't afraid to tell us a number, and we weren't left wondering how to help.
— Nikki Sprague and Amy Sprague, two sisters from Ashland, Wisconsin

Amy's Scale

Rating	What This Looks Like	Length
5	TAKE ME TO THE HOSPITAL ... NOW • It is beyond my control – I might hurt myself. • My thoughts are turning on me (I tell myself to find a safe place in my head, but then I feel unsafe there, too). • High worry. • Panicking fast – I feel like if I don't hurry up and get somewhere, I'll die. *There is a good chance you can't tell until I'm at a 5.*	(Varies)
4	• I'm very tired, but my mind is going so fast that I can't sleep. • I'm hyper vigilant – extremely. (So aware of everything around me; if I am able to go somewhere, I need to see that I have two exits to get out.) • I am very easily triggered. • I am starting to lose control over handling the triggers. • I feel almost manic because my thoughts are so fast and scrambled, and I'm terrified that I'll go to a 5. *At 4, I start to look for help, but I should've done so at a 2 or 3.*	Comes on really fast
3	• I am quiet. • I keep to myself. • I am very tired. • I sleep more, but I don't get solid sleep. *I pretend everything is fine.*	Longest
2	• Maybe a little quiet, because I am scared of something being off in my mind. • Something feels off in my mind. • I don't get solid sleep. • I still feel kind of like a 1, but there is something creeping in. *I don't talk to others about it.*	Can be long
1	• I look calm, OK. • I am willing to talk. • I am apprehensive about dissociating (always on the lookout). *Now is the time to ask me questions!*	Short (currently can be 2 weeks)

OK, I have another ...

I was working with a young man using a scale to address how his actions made other people think about him. He finally got the idea and started giving me examples of things that he thought were a 1 or a 2 or a 3. He then said, "Asking someone if I can touch them on the boob, that's a 4."

– Kari

The "Tried and True" Scales From the First Edition

A "5" Means I Am Screaming

Ned is a kindergarten student with ASD and obsessive compulsive disorder. He just couldn't understand about voice volume in the classroom. He loved to scream just for the fun of it and often talked in a really loud voice. If you said, "Ned, you need to talk softly," he would respond, **"Why are you saying that!"** (in a very loud voice).

We decided to compare volume to big and little and put it on a 5-Point Scale. The results were not immediate, and it took a lot of patience on the part of Ned's kindergarten teacher to keep working on it, but eventually Ned was able to recognize when his voice was too loud. To help prompt him, all the adults at school carried small 5-Point Scales in their ID tags. When Ned's voice got too loud, the adult would take out the scale and point to the volume he should be at.

At first this bothered Ned, and he would scream, "Don't show me a 2!" The adults were instructed not to respond to such outbursts, but to simply point to the number as a nonverbal prompt. Over time, Ned began to respond positively. The following story also helped Ned to "study" the concept.

When my voice gets too big

When no words come out of my mouth, my voice is at a **1**.

When my teacher is talking to me, I should try to keep my voice at a **1**. *No talking at all.*

Sometimes my voice is little.

Some people call this a **soft voice**.

This is when my voice is at a **2**.

I use a **2** voice when I am in the library. A **2** is like a whisper.

My teacher would like for me to try really hard to keep my voice at a **3** in the classroom.

This is like when I am talking on the phone, talking to my friends at lunch, or asking the teacher a question.

When I get upset, my voice might go to a **4**. This is when my teacher can remind me about using a **3** or **2** voice in school.

If I am out at recess and I want someone to throw me the ball, I may have to use a **4** voice to get their attention.

A **4** voice is pretty loud and I should try not to use a 4 in school or in a building at all. A **4** is sometimes called an outside voice.

Maybe a **4** could be used if I am at a ball game and I am rooting for my team.

A **5** means I am screaming.

I should only use a 5 if it is an emergency and I am calling for help. I should try to never use a 5 unless it is a real emergency.

It is important to know about how loud my voice is.

Some places actually have rules about how loud your voice can be, and all kids have to learn about voices.

My teachers can help me remember about my voice by pointing to the number on the scale it should be at.

They don't even have to talk about it. They can just point to the number and then I will know that I accidentally got too loud.

5 Emergencies

4 Outside; at a ball game

3 In the classroom; at lunch

2 In the library; quiet time

1 When someone else is talking at the movies

Voice Scale

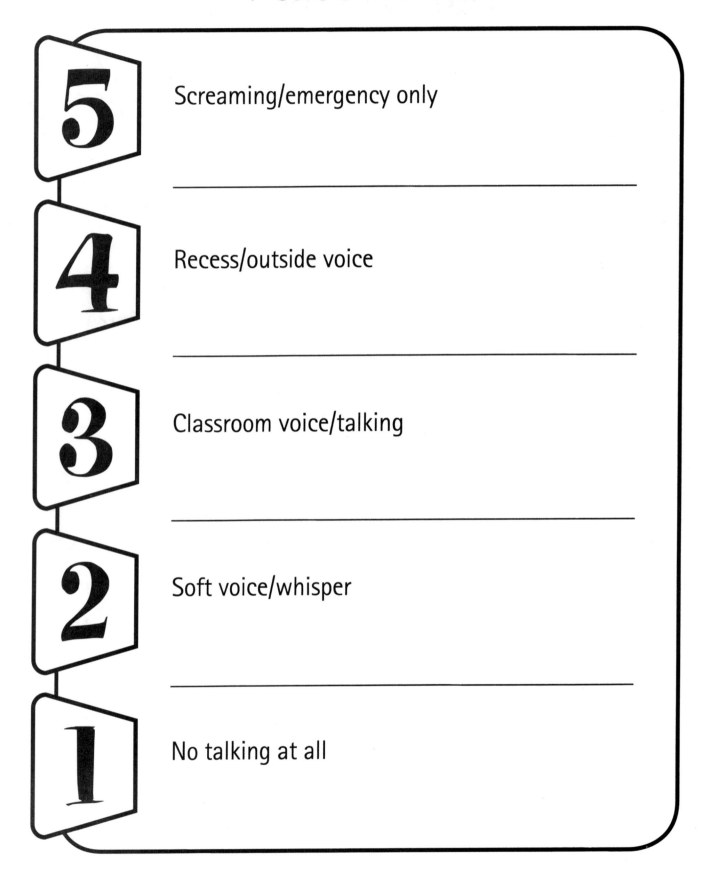

5	Screaming/emergency only
4	Recess/outside voice
3	Classroom voice/talking
2	Soft voice/whisper
1	No talking at all

When Words Hurt

Joey has ASD; he is in the third grade. He is very bright and likes to share his special interest in the Civil War with his teacher and classmates. Joey is fully included in the third grade and does well, with one exception: He upsets other children and his teacher when he says mean and hurtful things.

Joey often yells at other students when they say something that bothers him. Sometimes he is rude to others and calls them names. Not surprisingly, this hinders Joey's ability to make or keep friends. In fact, some of his classmates are afraid of him, and this is upsetting to Joey.

Joey thought that the only reason someone should be upset with him was if he actually hit or kicked the person. He thought it was illogical to get mad at words because words cannot cause bodily damage. One thing that has helped Joey understand the impact his words have on other people is a 5-Point Scale that illustrates various degrees of interaction. We used the scale to help explain the degrees of social interactions to him.

For example, he got very upset with a student who was sitting next to him and yelled, "Will you be ignorant forever!?" This was upsetting to the other student, who asked to be moved to the other side of the room. Joey was very upset by the student's response to his behavior. He couldn't understand why telling the truth would make her mad.

We explained it using the 5-Point Scale, with 4 and 5 behaviors being very upsetting to others. We also drew a cartoon to illustrate the social situation – with Joey yelling at the other student and the other student thinking, "Joey's behavior is at a 4. Those words hurt and make me want to move as far away from him as I can. Those words make me a little afraid of Joey because sometimes people who say mean things also do mean things." Joey asked if he could keep the cartoon in his desk and often studied it. We wrote a story about how words hurt to help clarify this concept for Joey.

The Incredible 5-Point Scale

There is no question that Joey is still confused by others' reactions to his words, but he is beginning to accept the fact that other people sometimes think differently than he does. Below is a copy of the cartoon that helped Joey understand the rating scale.

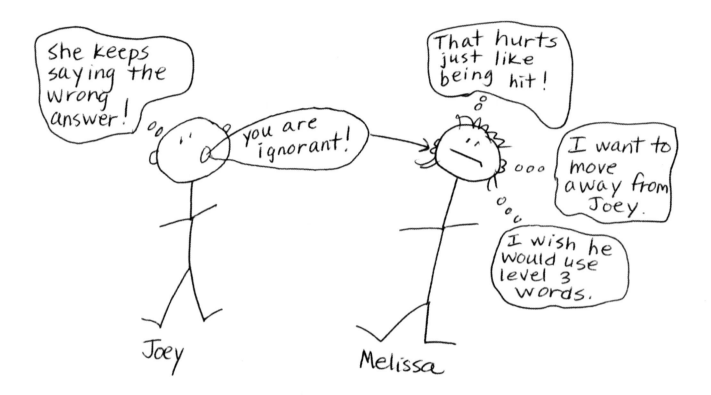

When Words Hurt –
A Story for Joey

Sometimes other people say and do things that make me mad.

Sometimes they give the wrong answer in class or break a rule, like cutting in line.

When people do these things, I get frustrated and before I think things through, I say things that are very mean.

When I was little, I used to kick people when they said or did things that made me mad, so I figured words were better than kicking.

Actually, words are better than kicking, but words can still be scary and hurtful.

When I say hurtful or mean things, other people may think I want to hurt them or that I don't like them.

When I say mean things, other people might decide to not be my friend any more.

My teacher can try to help by defining #4 words for me. I can write those words on my scale and try to remember not to use them when I am mad.

I can also keep a journal of the things that make me mad. Sometimes writing it down gives me just enough time to think about not using those #4 words.

The Touching and Talking Scale

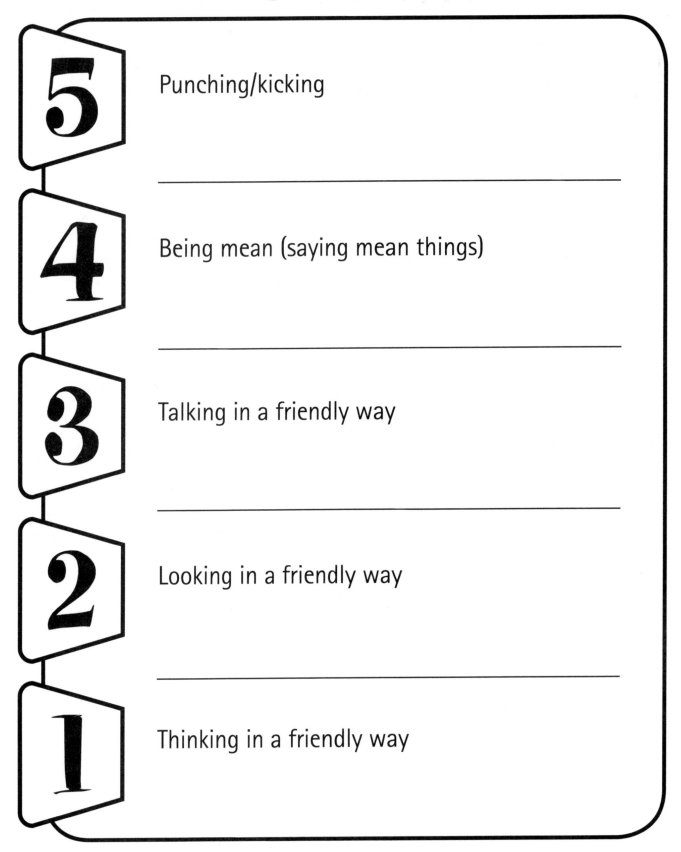

5 — Punching/kicking

4 — Being mean (saying mean things)

3 — Talking in a friendly way

2 — Looking in a friendly way

1 — Thinking in a friendly way

The Obsessional Index

Kevin is in the fifth grade. He has ASD and obsessive compulsive disorder. Kevin is obsessed with balls and will go to great lengths to find a ball and then throw it on top of the highest available ledge or roof. The ball-throwing obsession becomes a problem when he hurts others to get at a ball or when he runs through the school with a ball trying to find a high ledge. His anxiety over ball throwing is so intense that his thinking becomes illogical.

The following is Kevin's account of his ball obsession, which he reported to his teacher when she interviewed him as a part of a functional behavior assessment:

"I don't want to be obsessed with balls or balloons. It is a stupid obsession. I can't be the boss of anything. I want to be back to being a baby again. Maybe then I could start over. When I go to people's houses, I steal their balls, and that's embarrassing. No one in the neighborhood understands me. I hate obsessions. They make me mad. I really want to get rid of them but I can't. I can't do anything right. Every time I see a ball, I have to have it. I know right from wrong but this is just too hard."

The 5-Point Scale was designed to teach Kevin how to recognize his need for support in dealing with his obsessions before it was too late. On some days, he didn't even seem to think about balls; in fact, on those days his obsessive personality seemed to help him to stay focused on his work. On other days, he would think about balls but it didn't seem to bother him much. On those days, he was so relaxed that he could handle thoughts about balls.

Some days he just wanted to talk about his obsession with balls. If the adult with him told him not to talk about it, it often led to increased anxiety and acting-out behavior. Some days Kevin would come off the bus already talking rapidly about balls, types of balls, sizes of balls, and so on. We knew that on those days, he was going to need added support. This support often meant that Kevin did his work outside of the classroom to lower his anxiety about "blowing it" in front of the other kids.

Kevin had refused social stories in the past because he thought they were for "babies." Instead, we wrote him a memo to explain the new scale idea. Kevin loved the memo and kept it with him. He checked in with the special education teacher each morning to rate himself, and within a month he was accurately rating his anxiety about balls.

After we introduced the memo to him, there have only been a few days when Kevin had to work outside of the classroom for most of the day because his anxiety was high. Although he continues to have occasional rough days, he has not had to leave the classroom since we started the program.

MEMO

MEMO

To: Kevin

Re: When Your Obsessions Get Too Big

Sometimes having obsessions can be a positive thing, because it means that your brain is capable of latching onto an idea and not letting go. This can be beneficial for great explorers, inventors and writers. BUT sometimes having obsessions can be very upsetting and frustrating.

This memo is to inform you that I understand that sometimes your obsessions get so big that you are not able to control them because of the severe level of anxiety they cause. It would be highly beneficial for you to learn to tell the difference between when your obsessions are too big to handle and when they are feeling more like positive obsessions. One way to do this is to do a "check-in" three times a day when you consider your obsessional index. The first step is to help me fill out the following chart by rating your obsessional index on a 1-5 rating scale. Thank you for your cooperation.

Kari Dunn Buron

Obsessional Index

5   I can't control it. I will need lots of support.

---

4   I am feeling very nervous and will probably need some support.

---

3   I am thinking about my obsessions, but I may need to talk to someone about it. I think I have some control.

---

2   I am feeling pretty relaxed today. I can probably think about my obsessions but still do well in the classroom.

---

1   It is a great day! My obsessional personality is a neurological work of art!

The Incredible Home Scale

The home scale was created for Lindsay, a 10-year-old girl who has ASD. She tends to get anxious and stressed away from home, at the swimming pool, grocery store, church, and so on. As a result, when given a direction by her parents, she often screamed, kicked, and hit as a first response. This behavior was consistent whether the environment was unpleasant or exciting.

Lindsay's mother began teaching her daughter to rate herself on a 5-Point Scale: (a) before they left the house, (b) when they arrived at the destination but before leaving the car, and (c) then periodically while they were at the event or place. Finally, Lindsay's parents would have her rate herself prior to letting her know it was time to leave. This helped in preparing her for the transition to come.

Since it was important for her parents to honor Lindsay's rating, they carried small pads of paper so they could easily give her visual directives, such as writing out "Let's take a walk" when she had rated herself at a 3 and did not want anyone to talk to her. When she rated herself at a 4, her parents silently walked out to the car, and typically Lindsay followed to get away from what was upsetting her.

On those occasions when she didn't follow, Lindsay's parents felt that they had waited too long and that she had entered a 5 status. When Lindsay was at a 5, it was too late to move gracefully. Sometimes her parents opted to physically move her, but it was usually more prudent to just give her space. Giving her physical space often helped to calm her down, but touching her when she was already highly stressed usually resulted in uncontrolled aggressive behavior such as scratching and biting.

As Lindsay's parents learned to recognize subtle signs of stress, they prompted her to do a rating so that they could teach her to connect the subtle signs of stress with a 2 or a 3 rating. The long-term goal was for Lindsay to recognize those early signs of stress and excuse herself from a given situation.

Lindsay's parents learned that some environments were too stressful for her, and had to make some tough but more realistic decisions about their own expectations. For example, they wanted to take Lindsay with them to church, but realized that the environmental demands of church were too stressful for her and therefore made arrangements for Lindsay to stay at home.

When I Go Out

I love being at home.

I especially love my bedroom and the family room because all of my stuff is there.

Our schedule usually stays the same at home, so I almost always know what is going to happen.

Sometimes I go out with my parents.

Going out can be fun, but it can also be stressful.

One place I like to go is the YWCA.

I love to swim when I go to the Y.

When it is time to get out of the pool, it is often hard for me because I love it so much.

I don't want my parents to tell me to get out of the pool.

Another place we go is church. I don't like going to church.

I have to sit still for about an hour and that is too hard.

Sometimes I make noises and that bothers my mom. She keeps telling me to be quiet, and sometimes I scream out, "You be quiet!"

Yikes! The other people at church have a hard time listening when I yell like that.

My mom and dad get pretty upset when I yell at church.

One way to try and make things better when we go out is for me to learn more about how I feel and how to tell my mom and dad how I feel. That way they can help me when I start to lose control.

When I am doing something I really like (like swimming), I am usually at a **1**. This means I am handling it just great!

The Incredible 5-Point Scale

But my **1** can go to a **2** really fast if my mom tells me it is time to leave and I don't want to. When I am at a **2**, I am getting a little nervous.

When I am at a **3**, I usually scream things like "shut up!" I can let my mom and dad know about being at a **3**, and they will know that I need for them to stop talking right now.

Sometimes I am at a **3** for the whole visit, like when I am at church or when we go to my Uncle Ed and Aunt Sally's house.

I can let my mom and dad know that it is hard for me to be some place by telling them that I am at a **3**. If I am at a **3**, they can take me for a short walk.

When I get really nervous, I am at a **4**.

When I am at a **4**, it is important for me to go to the car.

My mom and dad always have special activities for me in the car (they are in my car bag). These might be my Little Mermaid figures, my squish ball, or my Gameboy.

When I am at a **4**, I need to think about relaxing. Closing my eyes and rubbing my legs and arms helps me to relax.

I should always let my mom and dad know before I go to the car. For example, I can yell out **"4!"** and they will know.

I can try really hard to bring my **4** down to a **3** by playing with my relaxing car activities.

I can handle **3's** much better.

Sometimes everything falls apart, and I need my mom and dad to help me calm down by taking deep breaths, not talking, and standing two arm's lengths away.

This is when I am at a **5**.

When I am at a **5**, I sometimes hurt other people and don't even know it.

I need lots of help when I am at a **5**. I usually need to take a nap after I hit **5**.

Keeping myself at a **2** is my goal. The more I work on this, the easier it will be!

The Incredible Home Scale

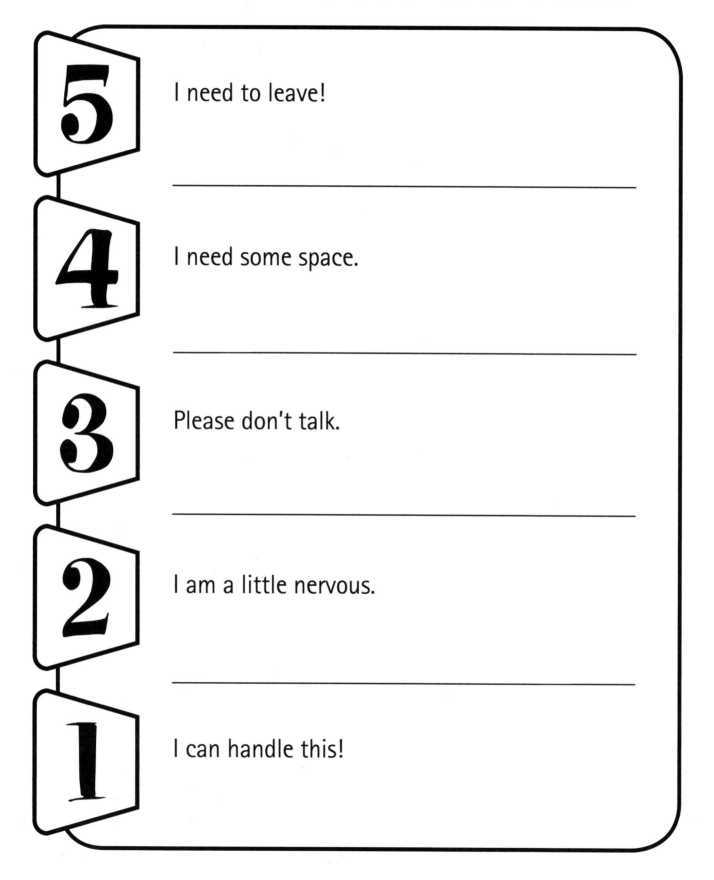

5   I need to leave!

4   I need some space.

3   Please don't talk.

2   I am a little nervous.

1   I can handle this!

Meeting and Greeting Others

Alex is in the first grade. He has ASD and is fully integrated in general education classes with support. He wants to have friends but has difficulty approaching kids appropriately. He often hits or kicks other students and gets into trouble. When questioned about this behavior, he denies ever hitting or says the other student deserved it because he was being ignored and that should be against the rules!

Recess is Alex's hardest time because it is loud on the playground and there is so much fast movement going on. He often gets very frustrated when he cannot get another student's attention. The following is a story written for Alex to introduce his 5-Point Scale as a way to help him control his frustration and approach students in a socially acceptable way.

Helping Alex Meet Friends

I really like to talk to other kids.

Sometimes on the playground I try to talk to other kids but they don't listen.

I get so frustrated when this happens.

Sometimes I say mean things or pull on their clothes to get them to look at me.

When I say mean things or pull on their clothes, the other kids say they don't want to be near me.

I need to remember to only use **2** and **3** behaviors when trying to talk to my friends.

2 and **3** behaviors are friendly words and friendly faces.

My teacher can help me by letting the other kids know I am trying really hard!

Meeting and Greeting Others Scale

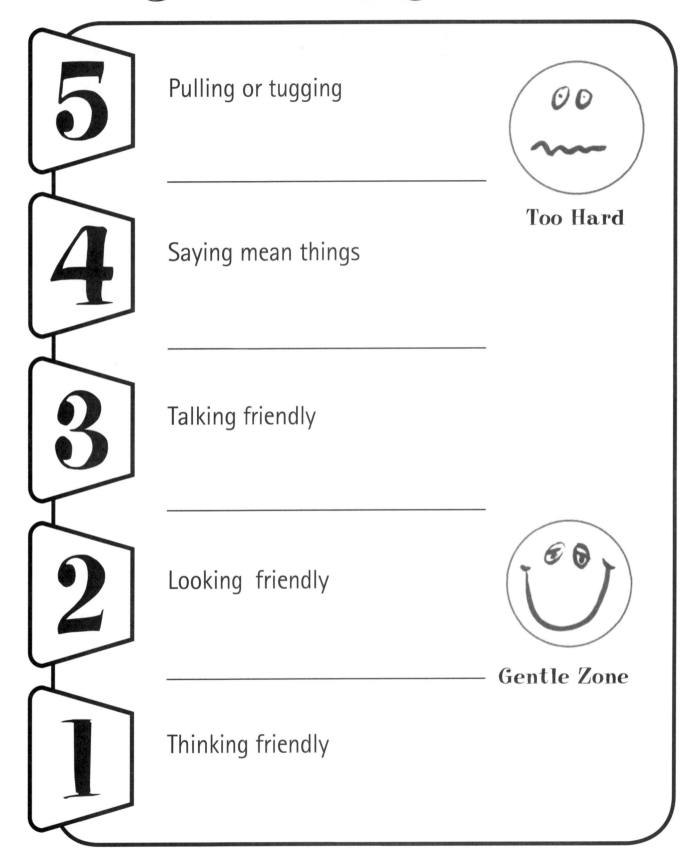

5 Pulling or tugging

_____

Too Hard

4 Saying mean things

_____

3 Talking friendly

_____

2 Looking friendly

_____ **Gentle Zone**

1 Thinking friendly

Control This!

Colton is in the fourth grade. He has ASD and has had problems getting along in school since he was in kindergarten. He likes to be in control and gets upset if he perceives that something is "wrong." For example, if someone cuts in line he may feel compelled to punish that person by kicking or hitting him.

Curiously, Colton's ability to control his aggressive response to others' behavior seems to vary greatly from day to day. One day he may not be bothered by another student taking two milks at lunch. The next day the same offense may be too much for him to handle and he may end up kicking the offending child. Colton's mother does not work outside the home, so she is able to come to the school and pick him up when he becomes aggressive.

The team decided to help Colton by using a 5-Point Scale to teach him to recognize his own ability to "control" his reactions. Using the scale, he started to check in with the principal four times a day to rate his level of control. If he rated himself at a 4, he would have an alternative recess (like playing chess with the principal) and eat lunch in the classroom with a friend rather than in the less structured and noisy cafeteria. If he rated himself at a 5, he would call his mother, who would come to pick him up before he lost control.

This program would not work if Colton did not like school, but he loved school, so he did not rate himself at a 5 very often. He was also very rigid and did not like to stay home because that meant a change in his day. He enjoyed recess and liked playing hockey, so he didn't rate himself a 4 unless he was very close to getting into trouble.

The program has not eliminated Colton's aggressive behavior, but it has helped him understand his lack of control. It has also helped the team realize that he needed more supervision and support in large social settings.

Learning About Control

Control is a funny thing. It helps to learn more about it and about myself.

It's okay to want to be in control. Being in control can make you feel more relaxed about things.

Sometimes I have lots of control. I am relaxed and feeling good.

I call this being at a **1**.

Sometimes I have some pretty good control. I can usually make a good choice when I have pretty good control.

I call this being at a **2**.

Sometimes I don't feel great. I may not even want to be at school. Maybe I just don't feel like talking.

On these days I don't have really good control.

I call this being at a **3**.

Sometimes I get up on the wrong side of the bed!

I am grumpy on those days and may not be able to make very good choices.

I wouldn't call this very good control – in fact, I almost don't have any control.

I call this being at a **4**.

Then there are those really, really bad days.

They don't happen very often but when they do, look out!

Sometimes I just lose all control.

I can't make good choices and sometimes I am in danger of hurting someone else.

This is being at a **5**.

It is good to learn about control so I can learn to be more independent, successful, and capable!

Name: __Colton_____ My __Control_____ Scale

Rating	Looks like	Feels like	I can *try*
5	Kicking or hitting	My head will probably explode	Call my mom go home
4	Screaming at people. <u>Almost</u> hitting	Nervous	Go to see Mr. Peterson
3	Quiet sometimes rude talk	Bad mood, grumpy	Stay away from kids (The ones I don't like!)
2	Regular kid – <u>not</u> weird!	Good	Enjoy it while it lasts
1	Playing hockey	A million bucks $	Stay that way!

What I Really Meant Was...

Emily is a fifth-grade student with ASD and Tourette Syndrome. She goes to a special school for students with severe behavior challenges. The program typically uses positive programming, but if the staff feel a student is becoming aggressive, a forced timeout – the stop-and-think room – may be implemented. Emily often complains that she has to sit in the stop-and-think room for not doing her work. Her teacher insists that Emily never goes to the stop-and-think room for noncompliance, only for threatening behavior.

We were asked to help create a program for Emily that would help her understand the perspective of others and the impact her behavior has on others, including her teacher. After observing Emily during a typical struggle with her teacher, we decided to meet with Emily and her teacher to discuss perspective-taking using a 5-point scale.

Emily truly did think she was getting in trouble for not doing her work. What seemed to be happening was the following.

When Emily refused to do her work, her teacher responded with an angry posture (her face and her body). When Emily perceived her teacher as being angry, she became defensive and engaged in verbally challenging behavior. If her teacher responded verbally to her challenges, Emily would start yelling. Often the yelling escalated to swearing and insulting remarks. At this point, Emily's teacher interpreted her behavior as one step before explosive and therefore directed her to the stop-and-think room. All the while, Emily did not feel she was out of control.

To problem solve this situation we first used a 5-Point Scale to define Emily's control, with 5 meaning out of control. Emily told us that if she was hitting, she was at a 5 but that if she was running out of the room, she was only at a 4. She said that she was hardly ever mad when she swore, so that was rated a 3.

When we interviewed Emily's teacher, she agreed that hitting was a 5. However, she thought that Emily's swearing was a 4 because it felt angry and intimidating. She agreed that Emily was probably still in control when she was just rude but not swearing.

We put the two scales side by side to illustrate the two different perspectives. We then drew a curve to visually illustrate Emily's level of anxiety. We used the scale to explain to Emily that her teacher had to predict when Emily would get out of control so that she could protect herself and the other students. We put the teacher's 1-5 ratings on the curve to help Emily understand that her teacher's actions were based on how she thought about what she was seeing and hearing.

The teacher and Emily agreed to try to "talk in numbers" in the future. The teacher agreed that if Emily swore, she would ask her what number she was at. If Emily said that she was at a 3, the teacher agreed to walk away and give her time to cool down. Emily also made cards with the numbers 1-5 on them and agreed to try to give the teacher a card when she was upset, instead of talking rudely.

The program had a dramatic effect on improving Emily's behavior as well as her relationship with her teacher, who became a wonderful advocate for Emily when the team began to plan for middle school.

Emily's Perspective

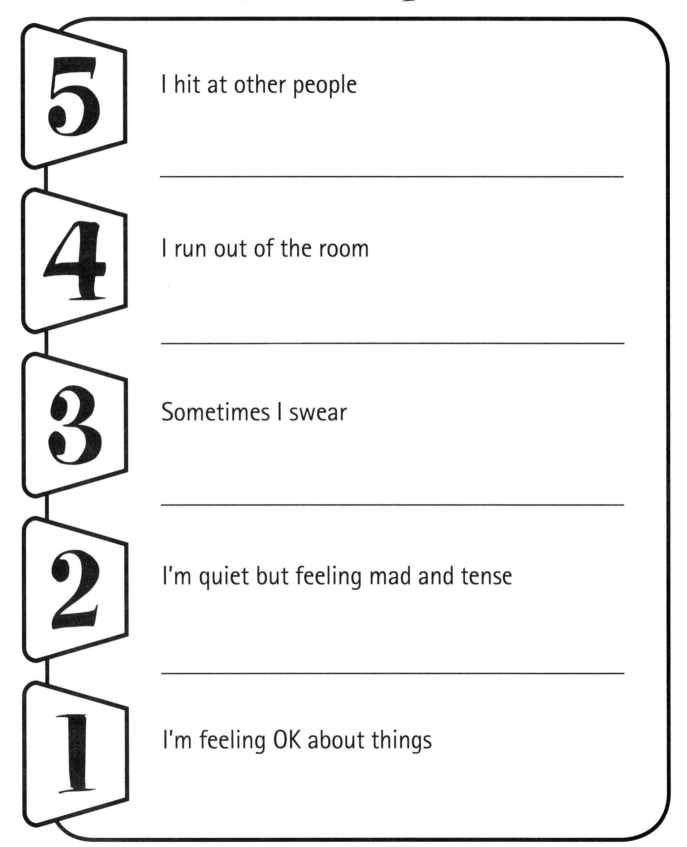

5 — I hit at other people

_____

4 — I run out of the room

_____

3 — Sometimes I swear

_____

2 — I'm quiet but feeling mad and tense

_____

1 — I'm feeling OK about things

Emily's Anxiety Curve

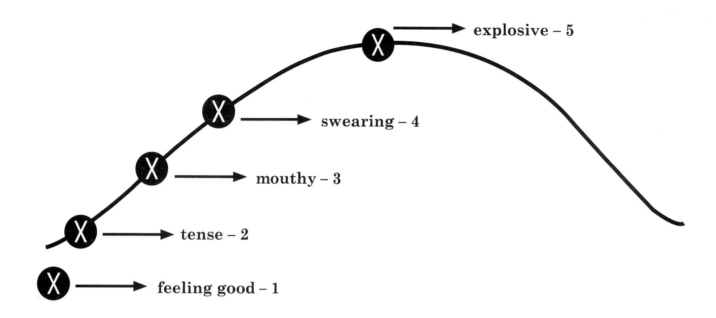

	Emily thinks	Mrs. Olson thinks
5	hitting	hitting
4	running out of the room	swearing
3	swearing	mouthy
2	mad/tense	challenging
1	OK	working

Emily goes to the stop-and-think room when Mrs. Olson thinks she is close to an explosion.

Meagan's Touching Scale

Meagan is a seventh-grader with ASD. She has recently begun developing physically and has started touching her breasts at school. The school team felt that she was trying to get attention because she often touched her breasts and then looked at her teacher for a reaction. This behavior was particularly problematic when Meagan was in the general education settings such as homeroom or lunch. Peers often became so uncomfortable with her behavior that they would move away. It seemed the more her teacher asked her not to touch herself, the more Meagan would do it.

First, we introduced some touching rules to Meagan through a Social Story™ (Gray, 1995). We discussed the approach with Meagan's parents to be sure we were in agreement about what to say and how to define the different levels of touch.

The school team agreed to read the story to Meagan each morning and to post her scale in her work area as a reminder. In addition, Meagan's teacher wore a small 5-Point Scale around her neck with her ID tag to prompt Meagan nonverbally when she touched her breasts. The teacher was instructed by us to touch the 2 on her scale to prompt Meagan to bring her 5 touch down to a 2.

Meagan's inappropriate touching behavior at school decreased by 40% within the first month of this new program. Besides, Meagan's parents reported that the scale was being used successfully at home. Her parents added a red 5 card to prompt Meagan to go to her bedroom when they began to get a sense that her touching was becoming inappropriate.

Touching Rules

I can touch my arms or legs or even my breasts.

It is important to learn about when I should touch my body and when I should not.

It is important to remember my touching rules.

I like to touch myself.

I like to watch other people's faces when I touch myself.

But here's the deal:

Some people feel uncomfortable when I touch myself in certain places of my body. We can call that touch a 4 or a 5.

Some people do not want to sit next to someone who touches themselves at a 4 or 5.

I need to try really hard to remember about the touching rules.

I can read my touching story every day to help me remember.

My teacher can post my touching scale in my office to help me remember.

If I forget, my teacher can point to a 1 or a 2 on her little scale so that I can try to change my touching level.

I can be really cool and follow the touching rule.

Name: __Meagan_____ My __Touching_____ Scale

Rating	Touch what?	Where can I do it?
5	Breast Genitals	Bedroom - Door closed
4	Thighs Bottom Inside nose	Bedroom or bathroom
3	Bare feet Belly	At home
2	Arms Legs Hair	Anywhere
1	No touching	Anywhere

When Using a Quiet Voice Isn't Necessarily a Good Thing

Larry is an 11-year-old boy with ASD who is very soft-spoken. He often waits for the prompt, "What do you need, Larry?" before he asks for help or directions.

The following scale was Larry's first use of a number- and color-combined rating scale.

For Larry, the topic of voice volume was perfect. His social skills group had been working on filling in the colors and numbers on the scale. We then assigned a voice volume to 5, deciding that 5 would be yelling. After preparing the group for what was about to happen and covering our ears, the facilitator demonstrated yelling. As you can imagine, the kids thought this was pretty funny. We then defined 1 as not talking at all. We practiced having our mouths closed and open. We practiced not talking. Level 2 was identified as whispering, and then we practiced whispering. Number 3 on the scale was defined as conversation, and we practiced talking so that our partner could hear us but not the entire group. Finally, we decided that 4 would just be loud, which might mean the person we were talking to would have to back away a bit when we talked. We also practiced that.

Larry, as well as many of the students in the group, seemed to need more than just the numbers, words, and practice to fully understand the concept of voice volume, so we added color and faces. This particularly helped Larry as he struggles with reading and number concepts and has difficulty discriminating between colors. Many students with ASD could benefit from using multiple visual cues (colors, numbers, pictures) to explain the concepts defined by their scales.

As Larry was coloring his scale, he stopped when he came to the number 5. He needed a red crayon but he did not ask. The teacher prompted him, and he whispered "Crayon, please." The facilitator pointed to the 2 and said, "Larry, you said 'crayon, please' at a 2. To get Wilma's (educational assistant with the crayons) attention, try saying it at a 3." He did, and promptly got the red crayon.

After about 10 more minutes of rating voice volumes with numbers and colors, a new teacher came into the room. Larry wanted to tell her that he wanted to check his schedule. Without the facilitator offering any other prompt, except pointing to the 4, Larry said in a very 4 voice across the room, "Diane, excuse me, check schedule, please." Diane responded with, "Okay, bring it over to me and we'll check." In the past, Larry would have whispered his request and then waited for someone to prompt him to initiate the interaction with Diane. The scale worked!

Voice Volume for Larry

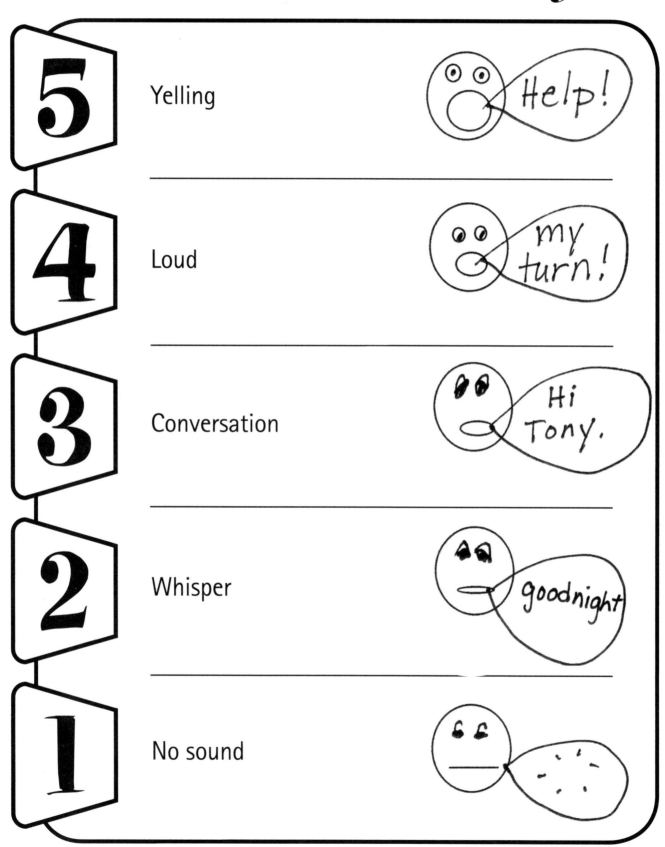

It Even Works with the Big Guys

The following rating scales were developed with and for young men with ASD attending a special high school for students with behavior challenges. We began working with these students one on one with their teacher present so that the concepts could be carried over to the classroom. In one case, we were able to have two students and two teachers work together. These two teachers voluntarily spent their preparation time learning how to implement rating scales with their students. The two boys knew each other and were willing and able to participate together during most, but not all group sessions.

The rating scales were developed within the context of the "group." That is, although we had some ideas about what social situations and rating scales to develop, the actual scales were completed during our meetings. A set of statements coined "Understanding My Feelings" (see pages 40, 43, 46) were used to facilitate dialogue and the development of the rating scales. These worksheets lent themselves to cartooning or other drawings by the students. When creating scales, it is imperative to listen closely to what the students say and to use their language. If they don't have the necessary vocabulary to label what feelings or behaviors they are describing, or what others see them do, come up with the vocabulary together.

The boys actively participated in identifying the specific rating values and descriptions. Their teachers also gave their perceptions. The results were remarkably insightful. You will see that some of the rating scales are incomplete. They are works in progress, but are very close approximations of examples of the boys' hard work. The rating scales were developed when the students were fairly relaxed and in a comfortable environment, such as an office, so that we would not be distracted by interruptions or inadvertently be joined by other people. The teachers and students then worked on applying this information to other situations and environments.

"I'm 6'2", Strong as an Ox – So Can You Tell Me Why I'm Trembling?"

David was referred to the self-contained high school program after being expelled from his home high school. He had broken several windows in the school cafeteria and the glass entrance/exit door nearest to the cafeteria. As a result, he had been to juvenile court and was placed on probation.

David identified his behavior as self-defense. "It was like my head was going to explode because of all the noise and confusion in the cafeteria. It's always confusing, and today there was a food fight. I had to do something to make it stop, I was afraid my head was going to explode."

The rating scale that follows does not rate David's level of anger, but his fear. David told us he feels afraid when he is "confused" so when developing this scale, we discussed things that we were afraid of, and David drew pictures to help him understand his own fear.

Understanding My Feelings by David

Scared/Afraid

My word for this is:
trembling

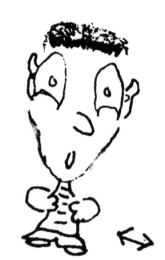

This is how I look:

This is how my body feels:

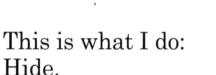

This is what I do:
Hide.

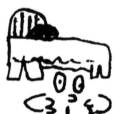

This is what I say:
"I've got to get out of here!"

Things that David says make him "tremble":
    "When I get confused."
    "When it is loud and crowded."
    "Catastrophes like tornadoes and earthquakes and war."

Name: **David**   My **scared/Afraid/Trembling** Scale

Rating	Looks/sounds like	Feels like	Safe people can help/I can try to
5	Wide-eyed, maybe screaming, and running, hitting.	I am going to explode if I don't do something.	I will need an adult to help me leave. Help!
4	Threaten others or bump them.	People are talking about me. I feel irritated, mad.	Close my mouth and hum. Squeeze my hands. Leave the room for a walk.
3	You can't tell I'm scared. Jaw clenched.	I shiver inside.	Write or draw about it. Close my eyes.
2	I still look normal.	My stomach gets a little queasy.	Slow my breathing. Tell somebody safe how I feel.
1	Normal - you can't tell by looking at me.	I don't know, really.	Enjoy it!

I'm Afraid I'm Going to Lose Control

Adam reported that he had difficulty managing his anger. He has assaulted others. Once with a tree branch. Another time he placed his hand around another person's neck as if to choke him. Both of these incidents happened while he was participating in an adapted recreation group social event, like a picnic or dance. Adam loves parties but is unable to manage his agitation, particularly if the event includes some sort of competition. In the above cases, Adam was highly distressed over losing a game. He hit the chaperone with the branch when he was told to sit out a game for using foul language, and he tried to choke his partner when they lost a game of tug-of-war.

Adam reported that the only time he was able to handle his anger during competitive games was when Lindsay, a staff person who used to supervise the adaptive recreation events, was there. Luckily, Lindsay was able to help create a scale for Adam. She said that she often noticed a change in Adam's body and facial expression prior to his loss of control. When she observed this change, she would prompt Adam to sit down and take a breather. This was not done as a punishment, but to help him regain his composure.

We developed a rating scale to illustrate how Adam "looks and acts" before he loses control to help increase his self-awareness. Adam's fear was that he did not have the skills to identify and manage his anxiety, and that consequently he would no longer be able to attend the social events.

The key to the success of this program was to inform all staff working the events that Adam was at risk when he was involved in anything of a competitive nature. All staff were given copies of the scale and directed to give Adam increased support near the end of game events. Adam himself was responsible for reviewing the scale prior to attending the events.

Although Adam continues to need support, he is beginning to learn to deal with the disappointment and frustration of losing. He recognizes some of his limitations and has opted not to play certain games if he is too worried about losing.

Understanding My Feelings by Adam

Scared/Afraid

My word for this is:
shy

This is how I look:
Mean

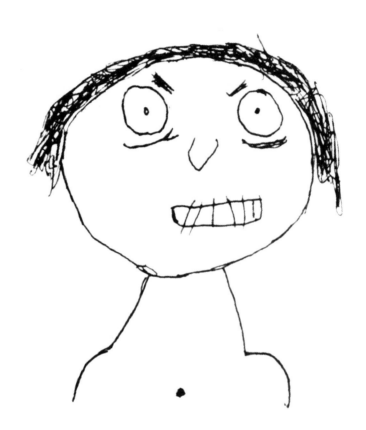

This is how my body feels:
Sick

This is what I do:
Hide. Hit people

This is what I say:
Swear

"Quitting sports makes me afraid because I don't want to quit. I'm afraid I might lose control at a game or a practice or whatever."

– Adam

The Incredible 5-Point Scale

Name: __Adam__   My __scared/Afraid/Shy__ _____ Scale

Rating	Looks/sounds like	Feels like	Safe people can help/I can try to
5	Swear Be mean Hit people Bite teeth tight	Sick Stomach turns Head hurts See too much, eyes wide open	(Work in Progress)
4	Swear Yell loud	Feel sick	(Work in Progress)
3	Walk around room	Can't concentrate Antsy	(Work in Progress)
2		My stomach starts turning over. A voice in my head tells me to do things.	Ask for or go for walk.
1	Put head down Hide Be quiet	Shy	Get reassurance from SAFE person.

"Take a Chill Pill, Sis"

Ben told his teacher that he said terrible things to his older sister and that he really didn't want to. He often engaged in verbal power struggles over doing chores, driving the family car, and so on. Frequently, interactions between Ben and his sister resulted in offensive language and even destruction of property. This is particularly troublesome because Ben's older sister, who attends a nearby community college, is often put in the position of looking out for him as his parents both work long hours and do not live together.

The following rating scale was developed when Ben's teacher shared with us that Ben was upset with himself over what he says and does when he is mad at his sister. He described a particular incident this way: "I had come home from working at my job for four hours. It was Friday. As soon as I walked in, my sister says, "You didn't do your chores. You have to before you can go out. And, I can't go out until you do!"

I told her, "That's not fair. I worked all day. Why don't you take a chill pill?" When she told me that I knew the rule about doing chores, I reminded her that last week she had let me go out before I had finished my chores.

This verbal exchange between Ben and his sister escalated to name calling on both sides, and eventually Ben left the house without finishing his chores. Before he left, he broke his sister's CD player and several CDs. He later came home and apologized, and offered to give his sister his CD player.

We asked Ben to fill out a feelings worksheet where he described the words he often uses, how his body feels, and how he looks when he is angry. The fact that he used swear words when filling in his rating scale was not judged as right or wrong, but simply as factual. (The use of these words was addressed later after Ben had gained some control of his destructive behavior.)

Besides rating his own anger, Ben also rated his sister's anger based on his perspective. Ben was limited in his ability to make a scale based on his sister's perspective, which is not surprising given the nature of his disability. Pulling the family into this situation proved helpful because Ben's sister and parents filled out scales based on their individual perspective. This information was extremely helpful to Ben, and it helped his family see how remorseful Ben was and how much he really wanted to work on his behavior. His parents also realized that Ben's sister needed more support in her interactions with Ben so that she didn't begin to resent spending time with him.

The process of change is often slow, and so it is in this case. Ben continues to struggle with his reactions to anger, but his destruction of property has decreased. He is working on role-playing possible frustrating situations and rehearsing reactions to help him cope better. He is also working on replacing swear words with other words so that he can eventually express his anger without intimidating or insulting his family, friends, boss, or other community members.

Understanding My Feelings by Ben

Mad/Angry

My word for this is:
Pissed off

This is how I look:
"How I feel I look,
but I really wouldn't do it."

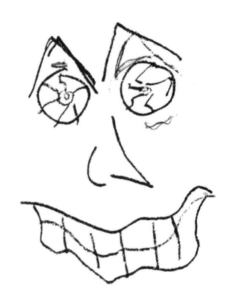

This is how my body feels:
"Like I will explode."

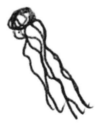

This is what I do:
"Throw stuff."

This is what I say:
*#!!@** #!@%/*##!!! ***#@//

Name: **Ben**   My **Angry/Pissed Off** Scale

Rating	Looks/sounds like	Feels like	Safe people can help/I can try to
5	Swearing Breaking stuff Clenched teeth Wide-eyed	I have to break something Feels like I need to leave Like I will explode.	Help me leave. Take a walk with me.
4	Swearing	Mad.	Leave the room with permission to go to a safe place.
3	Not talking Pacing A little swearing	Upset.	Go get a drink.
2	Not happy Keeping to self Still interacting with others	?	Talk to a safe person. Use deep breathing.
1	None?	None?	Talk to a safe person. Use deep breathing.

The Incredible 5-Point Scale

Name: __Ben's Perspectve__ My __Big Sister's Anger__ Scale

Rating	Looks/sounds like	Feels like	Safe people can help/I can try to
5	Bitching Yelling Screaming Throwing "you're grounded!"	Sick to stomach	
4	Ben says he doesn't know about "4" for his sister		
3	Ben says he doesn't know about "3" for his big sister		
2	Not talking Grumpy	Upset with another	Ben says he wishes his sister would leave.
1	Ben says he doesn't know about "1" for his sister		

Tell It Like It Is

The Tell It Like It Is Scale was developed for Richard, a ninth-grade student with ASD. Richard is partially mainstreamed but spends much of his day in a resource room. Richard often talks back to his teacher or the teacher aide when they ask him to do work tasks. His refusals include swearing. This usually invokes a reaction from the adult, which increases Richard's negative behavior. Richard is often asked to work in a timeout room as a result of these negative interactions. Frequently, his physical behavior escalates on the way to the timeout room (he throws chairs and desks).

The idea behind the scale was to take the control away from the negative behavior, create a program that was understandable to both Richard and the school staff, and teach Richard to recognize his rigidity and inflexibility. Richard was asked to rate himself three times a day (first thing in the morning, before lunch, and at 1:00 p.m.). The teacher wrote down the rating on his chart to remind himself of Richard's level of need. According to the ratings, Richard was set up at the group table (ratings 1 or 2), at his own desk (ratings 3 or 4), or in the timeout area (rating 5).

In addition, because verbal demands were typically met with resistance, the teachers began giving Richard written task lists (lists of 3-5 academic problems or tasks using the 1-5 terminology instead of verbally attending to any negative behavior). For example, when a student spoke to Richard and Richard yelled, "shut up!" the teacher told the other student that Richard was at a 3 at that moment and that he couldn't handle anybody talking to him. The teacher also reinforced Richard's ability to call a 3 a 3 when he was able to.

Richard later made a sign for his desk announcing to all which number he was at. This seemed to increase his ownership in the program and worked to help him communicate effectively with his classmates. The other students began enjoying rating themselves too, saying things like, "Bad night, I'm a 4 today."

Tell It Like It Is

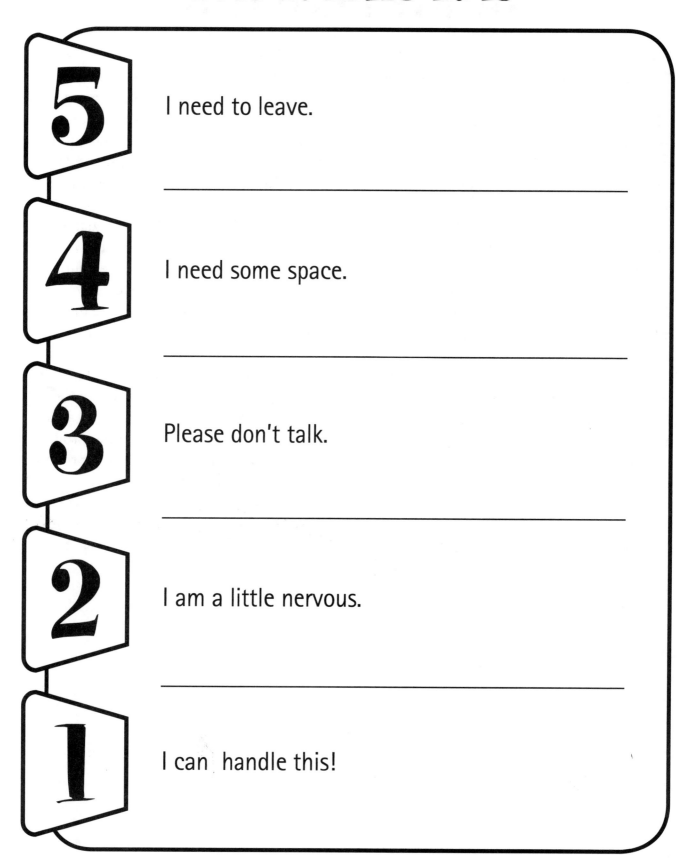

5   I need to leave.

_____

4   I need some space.

_____

3   Please don't talk.

_____

2   I am a little nervous.

_____

1   I can handle this!

One Step Forward, Two Backward

Sam was in our classroom about six years ago, when he was 12 years old, and we've kept track of him over the years, as he has of us. Sam has ASD and obsessive compulsive disorder. He has trouble with basic academics like reading, writing and math.

The occasion of his 18th birthday was a period of significant regression for Sam. Recently, with the assistance of his current teacher, Sam called us. He was particularly worried about his need to move into an adult group home and had been hospitalized for a medication change. He told us that he wasn't doing well. In the day and habilitation training program he attended, "not doing well" manifested itself in excessive sleeping, disinterest in work and, of greatest significance, harassment and taunting of other vulnerable 18- to 21-year-old students. Sam said he could not stop himself from the serious taunting and was worried about it. He also told us that he was not being physically aggressive.

Since we do not work at Sam's program or with him directly any more, this was a "create a rating scale right now" kind of a deal. This is the beauty of these scales. You can put them together methodically and polish them up or, as in this case, you can put one together on the fly. Sam's teacher had called us the day before, stating that Sam was not doing well. We were able to meet with Sam at his training program the next morning shortly after the start of his day. When we arrived, Sam was lying with a blanket under the sink in the nurse's office. We sat on the floor next to him, as did his teacher. It was important that the teacher was there as the rating scale would have to be polished up by Sam's teacher and others at his program since we would not be able to return to the site except to check in.

We wanted Sam and his teacher to identify whom he considered "safe people" at his program (people whom Sam perceives as understanding his disability and behavior) and "safe places" (places identified by Sam and the staff as places he can go to get away when he feels he may be unable to manage taunting in his current environment). All the significant people in Sam's life need to know who the safe people are and where the safe places are. Communication with team and family members is essential and should occur via a team meeting, phone calls, e-mail, or by whatever means the team members communicate with each other.

The following two scales were developed with Sam's input along with that of his teacher, right there in the nurse's office. The teacher agreed to work with Sam once a day to role-play, rehearse, and study the scales.

Sam and his teacher practiced what to do when Sam feels he is reaching a 3 on either scale. A 3 on the What Am I Saying Scale would indicate that it is time to find a safe place, away from people, to reduce the possibility of negative interactions and further escalation. A 3 on the Monitoring My Anxiety Level Scale would indicate that Sam needs help from a safe person so someone can assist him in regulating his anxiety. Sam needs an adult nearby when he is feeling anxious, which is also a time he is afraid of losing control and does not want to be left alone.

Not only did Sam learn to control his verbal taunting, but a year later he got a job doing janitorial work at a school program for children with severe cognitive disorders – something that would not have been possible if he had not learned to control his behavior with support from others.

Monitoring My Anxiety Level
A Rating Scale for Sam

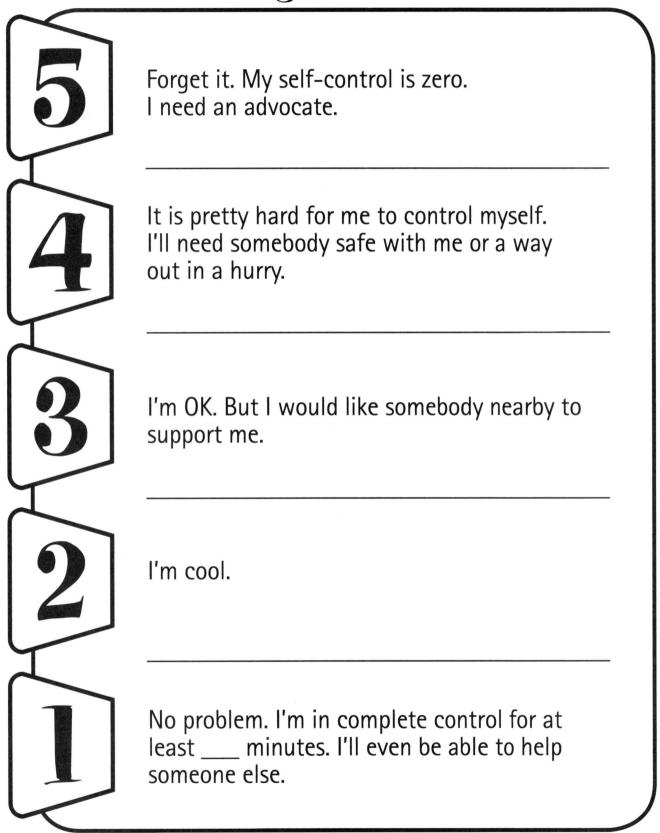

5 Forget it. My self-control is zero.
I need an advocate.

_____

4 It is pretty hard for me to control myself.
I'll need somebody safe with me or a way
out in a hurry.

_____

3 I'm OK. But I would like somebody nearby to
support me.

_____

2 I'm cool.

_____

1 No problem. I'm in complete control for at
least ____ minutes. I'll even be able to help
someone else.

What Am I Saying?
A Rating Scale for Sam

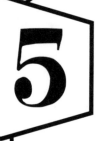

Taunting (for example, "I could kill you." "Go over and spit on the teacher."). [I need help.]

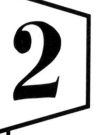

Negative interactions (for example, "I'm not going to do the work." "I hate this place." "Quit following me around.").

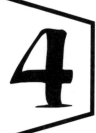

Short or no interactions, neutral. [Give me my space.]

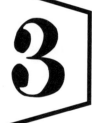

"Common" interactions (exchanging information about the weekend, asking what's for lunch, saying "hi."). [I'm fine.]

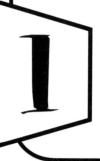

Positive interactions (initiated, "How are you?" "I'm glad I'm here." "You look great!). [I'm upbeat. I could help somebody else.]

Scales for Young Children

We have used 5-Point Scales successfully with children as young as three years old. However, we have met many teachers who prefer to use 3-Point Scales with their young students. They worry that breaking a concept or idea into five parts might be too difficult for young students.

Here are some things to think about when working with very young children.

1. **Ask yourself how we usually deal with unwanted behavior in very young children:** *We show them and tell them what we expect.* If a child does not seem to respond positively to this teaching strategy, he might benefit from a visual representation of what you are trying to communicate with your words and actions. The scale offers just such a tool.

2. **When deciding whether or not to use a 3-Point Scale or a 5-Point Scale, as mentioned earlier, remember that you are teaching a system for learning.** The idea of a system is the most important piece, so a 3-Point Scale is OK. However, we have found that some children on the spectrum have difficulty changing systems. For example, if 3 is the "biggest," the "most out of control," or the "fastest" today, how can a 3 later become an average level when using a 5-Point Scale? This rigid thinking could make it difficult to expand on the scale at a later date.

   An alternative is to use a number scale of 5 (with 5 being the biggest) but only use 1, 3, and 5 (see page 56). You are only breaking the problem into three parts, but you are introducing a system that allows for growth.

3. **Use favorite characters or objects as a part of the scale.** This helps build motivation for children to look at and attend to the scale during the teaching phase.

The Incredible 5-Point Scale

An example of a scale that keeps all of these issues in mind is the Pooh character scale for energy levels. The original scale looked like this:

Rating	Feels like:	Looks like*:
5	Too wild! I can't calm down.	Tigger
4		
3	OK – I can do my work.	Pooh Bear
2		
1	Too tired ... I feel like taking a nap.	Eeyore

* For copyright reasons, in this book we are not able to use the original licensed characters. For your personal and instructional use, please insert the child's favorite characters as appropriate.

After the child learns to identify these three basic levels of energy in her own body, you can add to the scale to teach more subtle levels of energy without changing the ratings for Eeyore, Pooh, or Tigger:

Rating	Feels like:	Looks like:
5	Too wild! I can't calm down.	Tigger
4	Distracted. I can't pay attention.	Piglet
3	OK – I can do my work.	Pooh Bear
2	Drowsy. I might need breaks today.	Owl
1	Too tired ... I feel like taking a nap.	Eeyore

Introducing voice volume is a popular scale in many early childhood classrooms. A 3-Point Scale can be used, as in the following example.

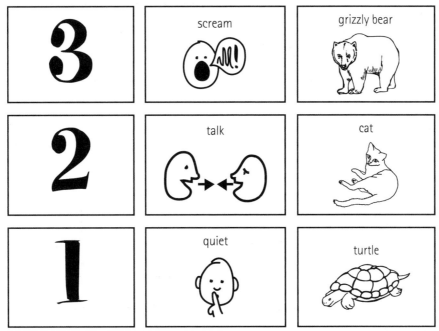

NOTE. Visuals are based on art made using Boardmaker (Mayer-Johnson; www.mayer-johnson.com).

4. **Write a story to introduce the scale.** Keep in mind, we read to our six-month-old babies, so don't worry about reading readiness skills. It is never a mistake to create literacy-rich environments for children. Here is an example of a story on voice volume that matches the scale above.

A Story About Voices

Sometimes it is time to have quiet voices.
Sometimes it is time to speak up so we can be heard.
Sometimes it is time to scream.

Quiet voices are whispers.
The words might come out slowly like a turtle.
Quiet voices are a #1.
It is good to talk at a #1 when you are in the library.

Talking voices are regular voices.
Talking voices might come out smoothly, like a cat.
Talking voices are a #2.
It is good to talk at a #2 at playtime.

Screaming voices are usually too loud!
Screaming voices might come out mean, like a grizzly bear!
Screaming voices are a #3.
Only use a #3 voice in emergencies.

Here is another example of a three-part voice scale used in early childhood.

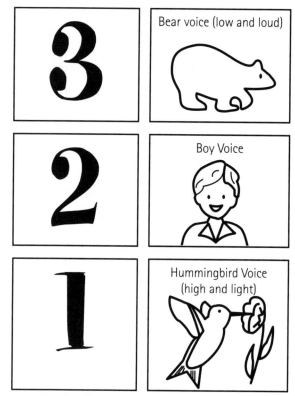

NOTE. Visuals are made using Boardmaker (Mayer-Johnson; www.mayer-johnson.com).

Caution: As mentioned above, if you choose to use only three parts, it might make it more difficult to expand later to a 5-Point voice scale where the #5 is a scream, #4 is a loud outside voice, and #2 is a whisper …

(The following educators assisted with this section by sharing their successful ideas:

Sarah Pedersen, early childhood special education teacher from Burnsville, Minnesota
Jason Backes, teacher from Minnesota
Amy VandenBerg, early childhood special education teacher from New Prague, Minnesota
Nicole Saatzer, early childhood special education teacher from New Prague, Minnesota
Kathy Ogden, teacher from Brainerd, Minnesota
Jan Stahly, early childhood special education teacher from Burnsville, Minnesota
Dana Randall, early childhood special education teacher from Burnsville Minnesota
Tara Tuchel, teacher from Stillwater, Minnesota)

5. **Involve the child whenever possible.** Any time you can arrange for the child to be actively engaged with the scale, you are sure to find it is well worth it. Try picture cards. Teaching a scale through the use of picture cards is a great idea. The child can then match the card to the "level" as a hands-on activity. The following is an example of how

this might be done (the child attaches with Velcro® the matching picture card (see below) on the right-hand side, where indicated).

5	Grrr! I'm ready to attack. I will make a bad choice.	◯
4	I'm starting to lose it. I might make a bad choice.	◯
3	I'm starting to feel irritated, but I can handle it.	◯
2	I'm feeling kind of funny but making good choices.	◯
1	I'm feeling SUPER! I can handle anything.	◯

(Idea from Jill Pring, a teacher from UpNorth, Minnesota)

Note. When using color, the color of the frame around a given card corresponds to the number of the same color. 5 = red, 4 = orange, 3 = yellow, 2 = blue, and 1 = green.

The book *When My Worries Get Too Big!* (Buron, 2006) was written for young children who have high levels of anxiety. The objective of the book is to teach a child to recognize different levels of anxiety and then to engage in a routine activity designed to calm his body.

The following scale was used in much the same way. Using the child's interest in dinosaurs, the three-part scale includes a section to be filled in by the child. The large arrow prompts the child to relax prior to reaching anxiety levels of 4 or 5.

My Dinosaur Scale
Sometimes I Get Mad

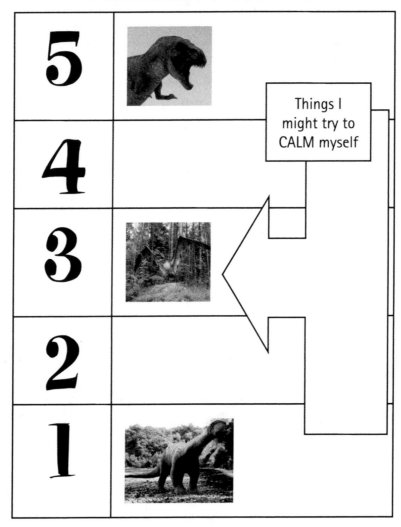

(Idea from Liz Delsandro, a speech-language pathologist from Iowa)

6. Make the number scale part of a chart, visually illustrating social behavior. The following scale uses high-interest trains to symbolize states of emotion, as well as possible outcomes and suggestions.

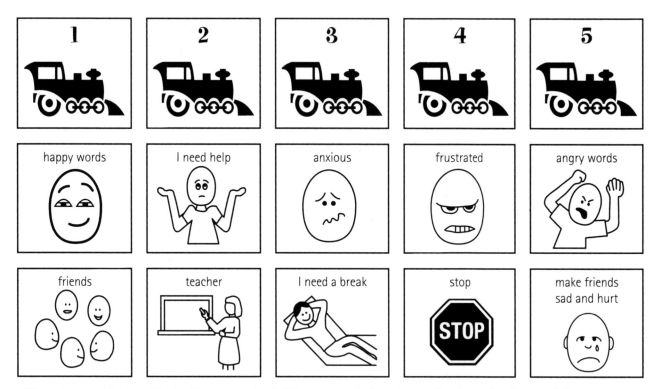

(Idea submitted by Amy VandenBerg, an early childhood special education teacher from New Prague, Minnesota)

(**Note.** In the above, the locomotives are presented in the five basic scale colors: 1 = green, 2 = blue, 3 = yellow, 4 = orange, and 5 = red)

The following scale was used with a five-year-old child who had minimal verbal expression. The child was struggling with his anger and frustration at home. The scale was used to help him identify each level of frustration using icons to illustrate number meanings; pictures of happy or frustrating situations; and pictures of ideas to try when feeling that way.

Thus, with the scale, the team made lists for caregivers indicating calming strategies that help and red flag issues that make the child angry. The lists may be expanded as new frustrations arise. The chart was used both to teach the child and guide caregivers.

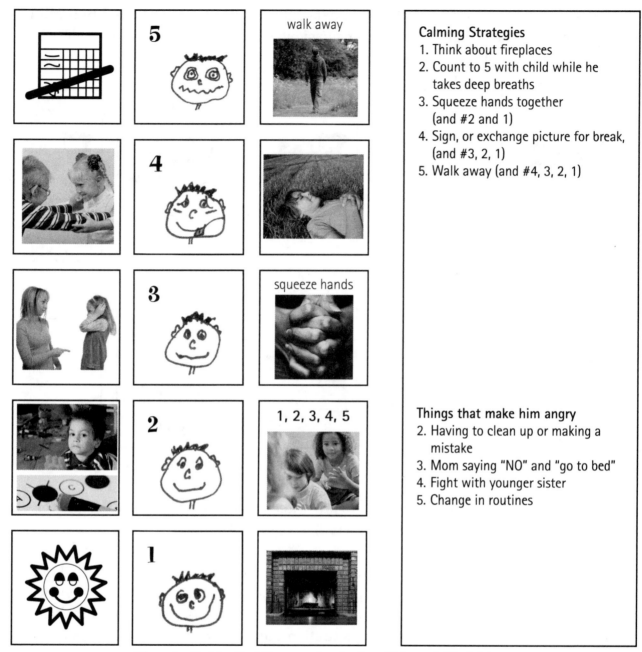

(Idea submitted by Staci Carr, an educator from Richmond, Virginia)

7. **Include high-interest themes and Power Cards.** High-interest themes have been involved in some of our all-time favorite scales and have proven successful through the use of Power Cards (Gagnon, 2001). The topics are best individualized, but if you want some practice, just take any popular cartoon, movie, or book and get to know the characters. In most cases, the characters have personalities that mirror our own. You can usually find three to five characters that can be used to illustrate the topic of your scale.

Examples of "themes" that have been used successfully with young children include:

- slippery fish (from the song)
- train cars (Thomas)
- Sponge Bob
- Disney characters
- Wild Things
- Curious George
- My Pretty Ponies
- family photos
- animals/pets
- food
- musical instruments

- dinosaurs
- Pooh
- Mickey Mouse
- Tom and Jerry
- Smurfs
- Wiggles
- super heroes
- Dr. Seuss
- Popeye
- Sesame Street
- Robby Blue Koala

One of the most common questions we are asked is how old a child has to be to use a scale. We hope this section has given readers enough good ideas to get started using a scale, regardless of the age of the child. Remember that the scale is used as a more understandable and systematic way of learning than the use of words. If the child you parent or teach is not responding to traditional teaching methods, try a scale.

5 Stars

Remember that the scale is only one example of using an over-practiced, predictable "system" to increase communication between you and your child or student.

Another example of a simple system is one Kari calls "5 Stars." 5 Stars is meant to be a visual representation of the passage of time, and is used to help somebody understand when it is time to stop one thing and go on to another.

Kari was working with a five-year-old boy in a kindergarten setting. Every day at group time, the boy would scream, and his educational assistant would take him out of the room so that he did not disrupt the class. Over time, he learned to scream so he could go for a walk. The teacher did not mean to teach him this, but this is what he learned. The 5 Stars system was used to interrupt the negative interaction pattern that had inadvertently been established.

The 5 Stars system consists of a cardboard strip with 5 or 6 squares (with Velcro on each square) and 5 separate stars (with Velcro on each star). The child is given the cardboard strip and told (in the case above), "We will be in group for 5 stars and then we can go for a walk."

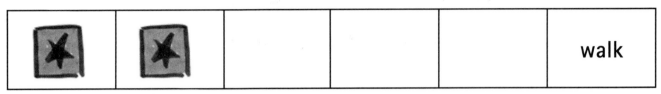

If you choose to use six squares, the sixth square is intended for a picture or word indicating what comes next (such as walk, recess, drink of water, etc.). The adult determines how quickly or slowly the stars are given to the child to put on the card, making it a more flexible system than a traditional timer.

> Please note that this is not a reward system. It is designed to be a concrete representation of the passage of time. The student does not "earn" or "lose" a star. In the above case, instead of staying in the group indefinitely or "for 5 minutes," the expectation is "to stay in group for 5 stars."

In the beginning, particularly if the student has already established a negative pattern as in the example above, the stars are given quickly so that the screaming can be pre-empted. As the student becomes familiar with the system, the adult can put the stars on at a slower pace, gradually increasing the time the student spends in group. It is the adult's responsibility to pay close attention to early signs of disruptive behavior such as blurting out, talking to self, or pacing so that she can successfully continue to pre-empt the scream while simultaneously trying to increase time spent in group.

The 5 Stars can also be used when you are nearing the end of a preferred activity. For example, if the student is playing in the gym and it is almost time to go and you are anticipating a negative response to your request to leave, try using the 5 Stars. Let the student know that you will be leaving in 5 stars, or say, "5 Stars and then gym is all done." Post the 5 Star chart on the wall and walk away. Gradually walk over to the chart and put on a star, possibly giving a verbal reminder of, "4 more stars and then gym is all done." When the 5 stars are on the chart, let the student know that gym in all done and it is time for classroom or whatever comes next. Remember to be patient, give the student the time he needs to process the functional and predictable system.

Scales for Students With More Classic Forms of Autism

We both started our careers teaching children with severe forms of ASD, and, in fact, first started using the 5-Point Scale with this population. Of the original scales, the following three were developed for individuals with extremely limited verbal skills: Lindsay's home scale, Meagan's touching scale, and Larry's Voice Scale (see pages 23, 35, and 37).

If you review these three scales, you will notice that Lindsay has a very long story. At first a teacher might worry that the words in this story are too much. However, it is worth noting that Lindsay's story came to school via her mother as a "preferred" activity. Her teacher put the story on her choice board because it seemed to relax her.

In our work with students on the autism spectrum, we have experienced a great deal of success using social narratives or Carol Gray's Social Stories™ (Gray, 1995). We believe this to be true, in part, because of the repetitive and systematic nature of the stories. Similarly, Lindsay's story seemed to please her despite being rather wordy. It sounded the same whether her mother, her father, or her teacher read it. The story offered information to Lindsay that she needed and wanted.

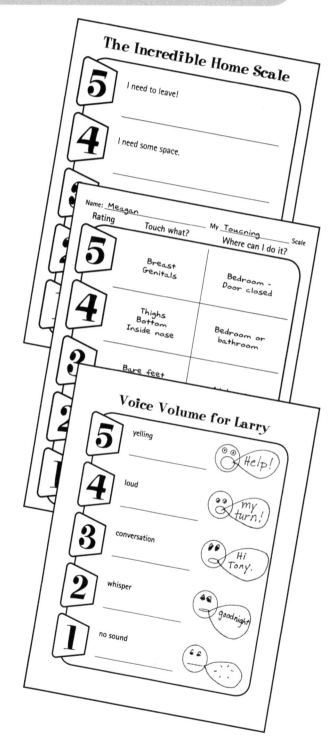

Concrete, Activity-Related Scales

Many teachers prefer to use three-part scales with students who have cognitive challenges because breaking a concept into just three parts is an easier and more concrete way to introduce the idea of using the scale.

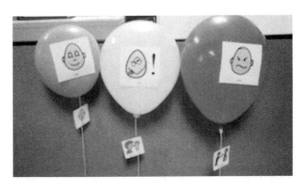

In this example, the teacher used actual balloons to visually illustrate three stages of energy and behavior. The smallest balloon illustrated a calm state, the middle-sized balloon illustrated a silly state of mind, and the largest balloon illustrated a mad state. The colors used are in line with the 5-Point Scale and allow the teacher to add a blue and orange balloon (to complete the five colors used in the original scale; 5 = red, 4 = orange, 3 = yellow, 2 = blue, and 1 = green) to the system in the future.

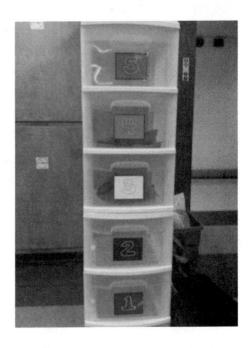

An activity developed to connect with the balloons involved taking pictures of the student in the three states and then matching the photos to pictures of various behaviors (laughing loudly, making silly faces, throwing toys, running, and sitting at his desk). Although this "scale" does not involve numbers, it is a system and, as such, it makes use of the systemized learning style.

Another way to make the scale more concrete is to add related objects and activities. One teacher first introduced the 5-Point Scale for anxiety, illustrating different calming activities that can be used at each level. A set of stacking bins were then labeled 1-5 and filled with various activities. The idea was that the child could rate herself and then choose an activity from the bin corresponding to her rating.

(Ideas from Jill Pring, a teacher from UpNorth, Minnesota)

Another way to add an activity is to have students color their own graph. This can be done on a regular basis, with or without support, depending on need. Over time, systems like the one on the following page are achievable by nonverbal students.

My Feelings Graph

By _____

Color one rectangle to show how you are feeling today.
Use the graph to see which level on the scale you feel the most!

1	**2**	**3**	**4**	**5**
Happy	OK	Nervous	Angry	Out of Control

(Idea from Nicole Saatzer, a teacher from New Prague, Minnesota)

Anxiety and Behavior Issues

Challenging behavior in learners with ASD has been linked to social differences or deficits. That is, when a person demonstrates challenging social behavior, he or she may lack the skills necessary to negotiate successful relationships (Aspy & Grossman, 2011; Castorina & Negri, 2011; Sansosti, 2010). It seems unreasonable to think that anyone *chooses* to fail at finding friends or leading a successful life.

One skill needed to create friendships or respectful relationships is emotional regulation. If a person cannot regulate her emotions, she is likely to demonstrate unpleasant or aggressive behavior when a social interaction becomes frustrating to her. Such challenging responses can be very upsetting for families, teachers, and peers.

If the person in question also lacks the ability to tell her side of the story, it makes things even more difficult. This cycle of ineffective social interaction can become damaging to the person and everyone who cares about her. This is a serious quality-of-life issue.

Typically, caregivers have the social skills necessary to create positive relationships. They are mature and flexible thinkers, capable of taking the lead in relationship building. If a person cannot successfully regulate his or her big emotional responses, the caregiver should take the first step. We need to create successful interactions, good days, and social enjoyment.

One way to begin this process is to use the Anxiety Curve worksheet. Max, a young man with ASD and Down Syndrome, offers an excellent example of how a team can use the Anxiety Curve worksheet to support a person.

In this case, the scale was used as a planning tool to assist caregivers in taking a closer look at Max's anxiety – what it looked liked and what seemed to make it grow. The process helped everyone to focus on how to avoid the anxiety in the first place. As a result, it was decided that the team needed to orchestrate a calm environment in order to begin creating positive experiences for Max.

The team's energy was spent focusing on how they could better "read" Max. Max seemed to be very reactive to the emotional responses of others. If the caregiver panicked, so did Max. The team members began to understand how their actions influenced Max's anxiety. They realized that they could offer a force of supportive calm or be faced with a force to be reckoned with.

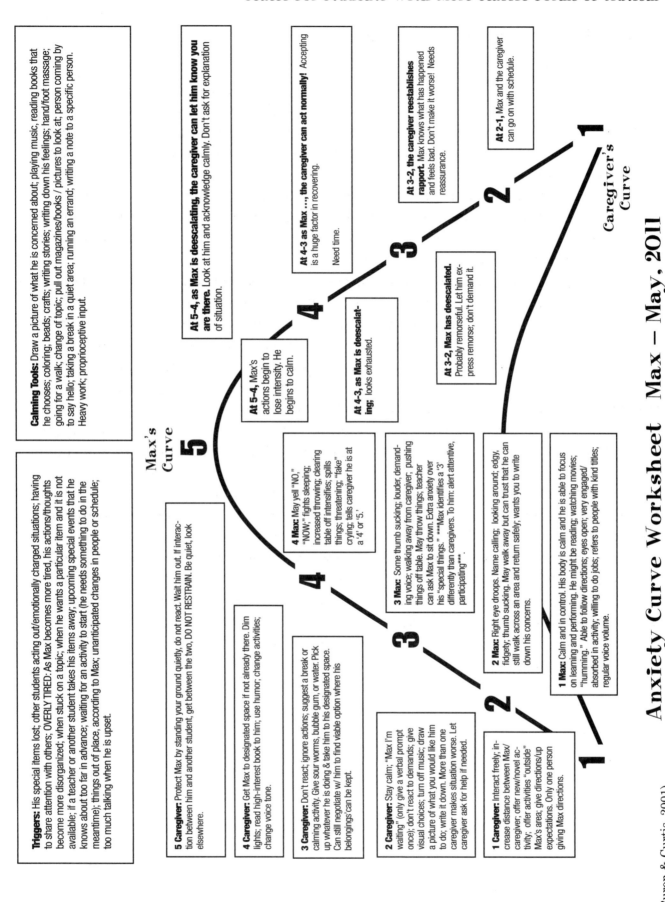

Anxiety Curve Worksheet Max – May, 2011

Max's Curve

Caregiver's Curve

Triggers: His special items lost; other students acting out/emotionally charged situations; having to share attention with others; OVERLY TIRED: As Max becomes more tired, his actions/thoughts become more disorganized; when stuck on a topic; when he wants a particular item and it is not available; if a teacher or another student takes his items away; upcoming special events that he knows about too far in advance; waiting for an activity to start (he needs something to do in the meantime); things out of place, according to Max; unanticipated changes in people or schedule; too much talking when he is upset.

Calming Tools: Draw a picture of what he is concerned about; playing music, reading books that he chooses; coloring; beads; crafts; writing stories; writing down his feelings; hand/foot massage; going for a walk; change of topic; pull out magazines/books / pictures to look at; person coming by to say hello; taking a break in a quiet area; running an errand; writing a note to a specific person. Heavy work; proprioceptive input.

At 5–4, as Max is deescalating, the caregiver can let him know you are there. Look at him and acknowledge calmly. Don't ask for explanation of situation.

Accepting **At 4–3 as Max …, the caregiver can act normally!** is a huge factor in recovering. Need time.

At 3–2, the caregiver reestablishes rapport. Max knows what has happened and feels bad. Don't make it worse! Needs reassurance.

At 2–1, Max and the caregiver can go on with schedule.

At 5–4, Max's actions begin to lose intensity. He begins to calm.

At 4–3, as Max is deescalating; looks exhausted.

At 3–2, Max has deescalated. Probably remorseful. Let him express remorse; don't demand it.

4 Max: May yell "NO," "NOW;" fights sleeping; increased throwing; clearing table off intensifies; spills things; threatening; "fake" crying; tells caregiver he is at a '4' or '5.'

3 Max: Some thumb sucking; louder, demanding voice; walking away from caregiver; pushing things off table. May throw things; teacher can ask Max to sit down. Extra anxiety over his "special things." ***Max identifies a '3' differently than caregivers. To him: alert attentive, participating***.

2 Max: Right eye droops. Name calling: looking around; edgy, fidgety; thumb sucking. May walk away but can trust that he can still walk across an area and return safely, wants you to write down his concerns.

1 Max: Calm and in control. His body is calm and he is able to focus on learning and performing. He might be reading; watching movies; "humming." Able to follow directions; eyes open; very engaged/absorbed in activity, willing to do jobs; refers to people with kind titles; regular voice volume.

5 Caregiver: Protect Max by standing your ground quietly, do not react. Wait him out. If interaction between him and another student, get between the two, DO NOT RESTRAIN. Be quiet, look elsewhere.

4 Caregiver: Get Max to designated space if not already there. Dim lights; read high-interest book to him; use humor; change voice tone.

3 Caregiver: Don't react; ignore actions; suggest a break or calming activity. Give sour worms, bubble gum, or water. Pick up whatever he is doing & take him to his designated space. Can still negotiate w/ him to find viable option where his belongings can be kept.

2 Caregiver: Stay calm; "Max I'm waiting" (only give a verbal prompt once); don't react to demands; give visual choices; turn off music; draw a picture of what you would like him to do; write it down. More than one caregiver makes situation worse. Let caregiver ask for help if needed.

1 Caregiver: Interact freely; increase distance between Max/caregiver; offer new/novel activity; offer activities "outside" Max's area; give directions/up expectations. Only one person giving Max directions.

(Thank you to Max and his mother, Katie Cookas, for permission to tell Max's story)

(Buron & Curtis, 2001)

More About Using Scales on Behalf of Individuals With Classic Autism: A Good Way for Caregivers and Substitutes to Know What to Do

Somebody who does not speak or even use his finger effectively to point will probably not be able to use a scale to rate his own level of anxiety or need for support. However, his caregiver can. Caregivers can use rating scales to determine what kind of support they think he may need to be successful.

As an example, take Joy, a young girl who is preparing to go to the media center at school. Joy is making happy, but loud, Level-4 sounds. She does not seem to be aware of or able to modulate her voice volume. The media center will tolerate a Level-3 volume when kids are involved in projects together, but as a rule, volume levels are expected to stay at 1 and 2.

What level of support does Joy need to enter the media center without causing a disruption? What level of support does she need to avoid being excluded from the media center altogether? The cue to the caregiver, in this case, the educational assistant, might be to wait before going to the media center until Joy's voice volume calms, or to wait until a louder voice volume is acceptable; that is, when the students are involved in some kind of group activity.

The librarian in the media center is happy with the educational assistant and Joy for not disrupting the class. The special education teacher is pleased that Joy was able to go to the library to join the other kids with their projects. The educational assistant is relieved that she successfully completed her mission of getting Joy to the library. Joy is happy to be able to spend time in the library. Everybody wins!

When using scales in this way, there is mutual agreement and understanding among caregivers (even when the case manager, teacher, or parent is not present) about what type of support a child may need. The child feels less anxious because she is not being told to "behave" when she doesn't know how. This, in turn, increases the student's trust in the caregiver.

Joy's Scale

5	Screaming. Calmly leave the media center now. She is not happy and needs something! Talk to most familiar staff. Please don't take Joy to the media center, even if it is on her schedule.
4	Yelling. Happy. Great for outside, parties, etc. Not OK for media center. Calmly wait for Joy to quiet down. It won't take too long.
3	"Ha," "Brrrrrrrr," uttered in regular "conversation volume." This is OK in the media center as long as kids are not supposed to be listening to a story. Find alternative media activities such as using the listening center away from reading circle; rejoin if noise becomes infrequent.
2	Very infrequent sounds. Variety of volumes. This is good. If short loud sound happens, may say "Oops" or "Sorry about that" to the media folks. The other kids don't care. The staff might.
1	Quiet. Fine for media center. But if Joy remains quiet for more than 15 minutes, check in with staff who know her best to make sure she's feeling OK. Quiet may be precursor to seizure activity.

Many individuals with more classic forms of ASD are not able to verbalize what they know, what they need, how they feel, or what they experience. Much of what we have learned about systemizing learning style, we have learned from individuals with higher functioning ASD, so sometimes caregivers of individuals with classic autism don't think it applies to their students. However, individuals across the autism spectrum, by definition, share the criteria area descriptive of autism spectrum disorders, that of **restrictive, repetitive patterns of behavior, interests, or activities.**

It is precisely these areas that relate to the hyper-systemizing learning style. We hope this section offers enough examples to help caregivers of all individuals with autism to begin using the scale.

More "Pretty Good" Scale Ideas

This section introduces nine additional scales with stories and details about how to work through difficult social concepts. We have also introduced three examples of how students can begin to "own" their scales by co-creating them. Having the person with ASD contribute to the creation of his or her scale can increase self-awareness and self-management.

Word Scales – What Did I Say?

Wyatt was nine years old and had been suspended from his elementary school for telling a classmate that he was planning to bring weapons to school. Wyatt was surprised and dismayed when the school administration took him seriously. He assumed everyone would know he was just kidding.

To help Wyatt understand how his words made other people think, his teacher created a 5-Point Scale of word categories. She decided on the following rating:

- #1 – words that made other people think that Wyatt was nice and called these "sweet words";
- #2 – words that didn't bother other people but that weren't particularly friendly either; she called these "just fine words";
- #3 – words that would likely hurt someone's feelings; she called them "hurtful words";
- #4 – words that made other people think that Wyatt was mean, so these were called "angry words";
- finally, #5 – words that made other people feel that he was dangerous. These were the worst possible words.

Wyatt's teacher introduced the scale to Wyatt using the following story.

The Power of Words

The words we say do make a difference. Even if you don't feel like you are a threat to other people, your actions and words might make other people feel that you are.

Other people can't read your mind, so they have to listen to your words and guess what you are thinking about.

It is important to study your Word Scale and think about the words you say out loud.

Even if you think #4 and #5 words, it is best to keep them inside your think bubble.

When people hear #4 and #5 words, they might think you are dangerous. They will have to do something.

Study your scale and remember: ***Don't Pop Your Think Bubble!***

(Emily Peck, a camper and fifth-grade student, first coined the phrase *Don't Pop Your Think Bubble*)

Wyatt's Word Scale

5	**The worst possible words.** These are threatening words. These words make people think you are going to hurt them. These words are against the law! Saying you are going to kill someone or bring a gun to school are examples of #5 words.
4	**Angry words.** These are words that people say when they are very angry. They are usually swear words. Saying a swear word could get you in trouble at school. Using swear words is a bad habit, so be careful!
3	**Hurtful words.** These are words that make other people feel sad or upset. They might be rude words about how someone looks, or they may be teasing words. These words make other people feel uncomfortable around you. It is hard to make many friends when you use hurtful words. Telling someone they are fat is an example of a #3 word.
2	**"Just fine" words.** These words feel pretty good to other people. "Just fine" words are everyday words like "hi" or "see you later." People feel good when you use these social words. These are words that make other people feel comfortable.
1	**Sweet words.** These are words that can make someone else feel good about himself. Sweet words are compliments like, "I like your hat" or "what a nice drawing." We say these words to people because we want to make them feel good. Using sweet words is one of the best ways to make friends.

Congratulations to Graciela Corella, a teacher in El Paso, Texas, who added to the lesson by pointing out that #1/#2 words were assertive and #3/#4 and #5 words were aggressive, thereby adding even further clarification for her students.

Here is another example of a "word" scale. This one addresses both the words and the tone/volume.

5	**Violent words.** Swearing words. Screaming words. These words mean that I have lost control. Words at the #5 level make other people think that I am dangerous.
4	**Scary words.** These are really loud words. When I use these words, people think that I might want to hurt them. These are not friendly words. It is hard, but it is really important to learn how to keep my voice volume from getting to a #4.
3	**Abrupt words.** These are words that seem to come out of nowhere. When someone says "hi" to me in the hallway and I wasn't expecting it, it can be a #3. Abrupt words might make me yell out, "shut up!" or "go away!" This usually means I can't think of anything else to say. I can try to just say "hi."
2	**Friendly words.** These are words that go gently into other people's ears. Friendly words make people feel good inside. Usually, the more friendly words a person uses at school, the easier it is to make friends. Kids and teachers all love friendly words.
1	Tiny words. These are words that are too tiny for the moment. This would be like when the teacher asks me a question and I am a little worried about saying the wrong thing, so I say it really softly. Sometimes people say #1 talk is like mumbling. This is reasonable since it can be scary to answer questions in group.

When Is Too Close ... Too Close? Scale

Carter was an eighth-grade boy who had recently started to hug and kiss his teachers. At first this seemed innocent and sweet because Carter had previously not shown much emotion towards his teachers. However, as time went on, the adults began to worry that Carter did not seem to have any boundaries regarding his hugs and kisses. He was used to hugging and kissing his mother as a way of showing affection, but now he started kissing less familiar adults and people who were obviously uncomfortable with that level of intimacy.

Early attempts to teach replacement behaviors (giving high-fives) and distinguishing between home and school behavior not only didn't work but actually caused an increase in the behavior. Carter started following the teachers around the classroom making kissing noises, calling their names, and blowing kisses.

The team determined that Carter wanted to be friendly but did not understand how this particular behavior was making other people feel. They designed a scale to honestly and visually map out the different levels of interpersonal behavior. The scale was created, printed, and introduced to Carter in a 1:1 session. In this scale, the team decided to make the #2 green to emphasize the number they wanted him to focus on. After only one review of the scale, Carter seemed to get it. He started using high-fives that same day!

It has been a year since the scale was introduced, and Carter continues to use high-fives to greet people outside of his family. He was having a particularly rough day a few months ago, and his teacher felt that he needed a hug. She asked his permission to hug him; he said yes, and they hugged. When the crisis was over, Carter continued to give high-fives with no sign of reverting back to his old pattern of indiscriminate hugs and kisses.

(Story comes from Tonya Lee, a teacher from Fridley, Minnesota)

When Is Too Close … Too Close? Scale

Rating	What does this look like?	How does it make other people feel?	What is a likely outcome?
5	Unwanted touching and kisses.	Violated!	This is not good. Staff will feel unsafe working with you, and other students will need to report this behavior to an adult. This is against the law for adults!
4	Following someone around and acting like you want to kiss them.	Very uncomfortable. Unsafe.	This can make people afraid of you. It is unlikely anyone would feel safe being around you.
3	Blowing kisses to someone outside of your family or telling them you want to touch and kiss them; staring at someone for long periods of time.	Uncomfortable and weird. This is confusing to most people.	People might not know if you are nice or mean. Therefore, they might decide to stay away from you.
2	High-fives; saying good morning; smiling at another person.	Good. These interactions make others feel good about being with you.	Making friends; favorite staff wanting to work with you. People wanting to sit next to you.
1	No interaction at all.	Others might think you don't like them.	It would be hard to make friends this way.

Having Our Say — Self-Advocacy Scales

Developing and enhancing self-advocacy skills can take many forms. The scales introduced in this story represent the basics of self-advocacy. Using these scales, the person is able to give input into what he will be doing, and even evaluate the activity after it is finished. The following examples were used in a group setting and are less personalized than the previous scales. The scales are used to reflect each group member's opinion and are used in an ongoing systematic way.

The scales were developed for a middle school social understanding class made up of four reluctant participants. The goal of the class was to provide direct instruction in social skills and concepts. To assist in generalization, the students' teachers and/or instructional aides were ask to participate in the class and model skills in other settings in the school throughout the week.

Because the students were not eager to attend or work on these skills, an "adversarial" relationship was beginning to develop between the students and the staff. The hope was that the self-advocacy scale activities would promote more positive and respectful relationships.

The Opinion Scale was developed as a survey for the students to fill out days prior to the actual class. The scale was meant to give the students a forum, with a trusted adult, for saying or writing what they thought. This offered a structured way for the students to suggest the content of the social lessons. Since the Opinion Scale was used prior to class, the upcoming topic was then announced in advance of the actual class.

The Check-out Scale was displayed on a Smart Board at the end of each class period. This scale wasn't about the students' emotional levels but about the quality of the lesson. When this scale was first introduced, all four students agreed that the first lesson was "better than they expected."

These rating scales helped to promote positive rapport between the students and educational staff. The approach seemed to empower the students and give them a sense of control. A cooperative tone was established between all group members, and a good dose of humor accompanied many of the "reviews" and suggestions.

Opinion Scale

Topic: Do you want to come to Social Understanding Class next Tuesday? We will be watching a biography about Albert Einstein and some problems he had with social skills.

Circle your rating.

5   **4**   **3**   **2**   **1**

Sounds good   maybe   No way!

Why? _____

_____

Do you have an idea for something we should do during Social Understanding Class?

What? _____

_____

Check-out Scale

This Social Understanding Class was . . .

5 – Great! One of the best, because:

4 – Better than I expected, because:

3 – As I expected (good, middle, bad), because:

2 – Not as good as I expected, because:

1 – Terrible. One of the worst, because:

Here Is Another Great Group Idea

The students in this group had previously been introduced to the Anxiety Scale, and students had created their own scale using their own words to define each level. The teacher was then able to use the learned routine to send out this reminder, incorporating language from the scale that everybody was familiar with.

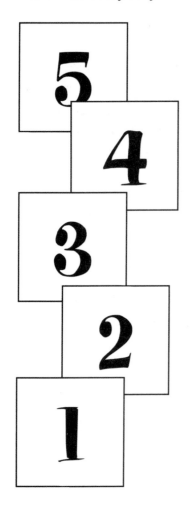

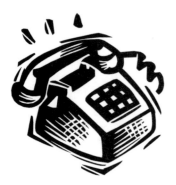

- Memo -

To: Social Thinkers Groups
From: Mrs. Pring

We just wanted to take the time to remind you of the importance of using your 5-Point Scale.

Remember, the 5-Point Scale is meant to help you understand your anxiety better, and is an easy system that allows you to self-monitor your own feelings.

In order to successfully use your 5-Point Scale, it is important to remember that when you are at a **3**, it's time to use your help lines. If you wait until you are at a **4** or a **5**, it is too late!

Your **help lines** are people close to you who are around to help remind you to use your scale. Your help lines are also the strategies on your scale.

At school, your help lines are:
     – Mrs. Pring
     – Mrs. Johnson
     – Mr. Berg
     – _____
     – _____

At home, your help lines are:
     – your parents
     – your siblings
     – other relatives

Using your **help lines** will ensure that you can come to school and have an awesome day!

Thank you for your attention to this matter.

(Idea from Jill Pring, a teacher from UpNorth, Minnesota)

Personal Speed Scale

The Personal Speed Scale was developed for two third-grade boys who often ran in the hallway. One of the boys, Obdee, had ASD; the other boy, Austin, did not. After coming in from outdoor recess, their habit was to run full speed toward their classroom door, and at about 20 feet out, slide on their knees, seeing who could get the closest to the door.

Their timing needed to be pretty accurate as the teacher returned to her room when recess ended. Obdee did not understand that this subtle part of the situation was required so as not to be caught. One day, as Austin was about to go to his knees, he saw the teacher at the classroom door and stopped immediately. Obdee, on the other hand, continued as always, thrilled that his classmate had given up and that he, therefore, was sure to win the contest.

Obdee was shocked when he got into trouble for running and sliding in the hallway. He told the teacher that Austin had been running too and thought the teacher was being unfair when Austin did not get into trouble.

In this case, the scale was made after Obdee got into trouble. His special education teacher used Obdee's misfortune to develop the scale as a way to work on self-management based on the following critical factors: where you are, who you are with, who might see you, and what you are doing.

The teacher used cartooning (Gray, 1995) to process the incident with Obdee, including thinking and talking bubbles to help him understand how other people think about things they see. She included the perspectives of his peers and his third-grade teacher.

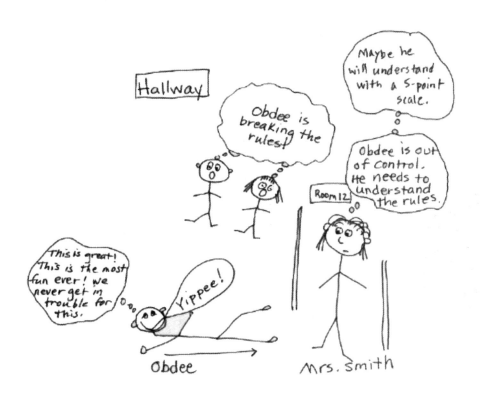

After the review with cartoons, the teacher developed a personal speed scale with Obdee. Obdee helped by labeling the speeds (snail, race car, etc.) and determining when different speeds were okay and not okay. Next, Obdee's whole third-grade class went over the scale with the teacher. His classmates also had an opportunity to contribute to the scale, adding ideas about what speed should be used for a fire drill, school dismissal, and the track and field day.

This scale can easily be adapted for other "sometimes breaking the rule" topics such as passing notes to a classmate, and for older individuals, using social media, such as Facebook or texting during work time, or staying on a break a few extra minutes.

Personal Speed Scale

Rating	Speed	OK	Not OK
5	Indy 500! Running full speed!		
4	Running or jogging		
3	Fast walking or skipping		
2	Walking		
1	Walking very slowly		

In this example, Obdee helped to name the speeds, and then he and his teacher filled in the boxes indicating where each speed is OK and not OK based on the following conditions:

- Where am I? Is this an OK place for this speed?
- Who am I with? Will this person be upset with this speed?
- What am I doing? Is it work time? Is it play time?
- Who can see me? Does it matter if certain people can see me?

Two More Examples of Speed Scales

These scales used graphics to define the varying speed levels. The first scale defines each level while the second example labels each action.

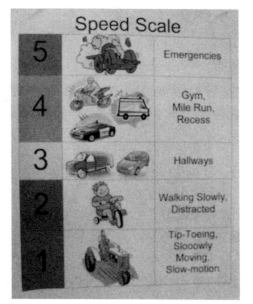
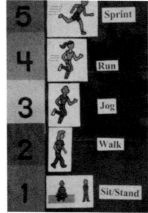

(Examples submitted by Chris Reano, a teacher from Bloomington, Minnesota)

Sensory Scales

We have had success creating scales about food, taste, sounds, and places. Many learners on the autism spectrum become overwhelmed by sensory issues. An example might be an environment scale, where a #1 would be a place so comfortable that someone could sleep there; a #2 might be a nice place; a #3 might be an exciting place (fun to be in but not relaxing); a #4 might be a place that makes the person feel uncomfortable; and #5 might be a place the person hates and avoids at all cost.

Once you develop an environmental scale, you can make picture cards of all the different places the person might frequent at school, in the neighborhood, with family, or at work. The person can then match the cards to the rating as a way of giving feedback.

It is important to then create a program that shows respect for this input. For example, if the gym is rated at a #5, it is essential that the educational team evaluate the possible reasons why that might be. Is it too unstructured? Are there unmonitored times where teasing might happen? Is the student confused by the expectations? Once the environment has been evaluated, supports can be put in place to make it easier for the person to function in that particular setting.

This activity was first developed as an anxiety-level labeling task (Buron, 2007), but it has since gained popularity as a method of getting the individual's perspective regarding various sensory sensitivities. Sensory challenges are very individualized. Not all people on the spectrum are bothered by touch, noise, or taste and, therefore, require different levels of support depending on their individual issues. For example, if a child is highly anxious in the

The Incredible 5-Point Scale

lunchroom, it might be due to the smells, the noise level, the number of moving bodies, and/or the unpredictable nature of energetic peers. Similarly, if an adult with ASD is upset in a particular environment, like a workplace, multiple reasons involving the senses could be contributing to her anxiety.

The following example was inspired by an activity we saw on YouTube. In the video, a researcher is working with a young girl, asking her to put pictures of various foods into the square that best describes how she feels about it.

Rating	How I Feel It	What I Can Do	Example of This Kind of Food
5	This is disgusting! I will never eat it!	Say, "No thank you."	
4	I don't want to eat this.	Put it to the side of the plate. Offer it to someone else.	
3	I will eat this.	OK.	
2	I like this!	Glad we are having it for lunch today.	
1	I love eating this!! One of my very favorite things to eat!!	I look forward to this. I would like it every day!	

(Based on Mark de Sagun, YouTube demonstration)

This Is Not a Competition! Scale

Ned, a fourth grader, had a strong desire to win. He seemed to have intense anxiety associated with almost any interpersonal situation, and that anxiety became an urge to "win." This was the case whether it was "winning" at being first in line, "winning" at being first to get a paper passed back, "winning" at being first on the bus, or "winning" at a game at recess.

It seemed obvious to the educational team that Ned was lacking some basic understanding of the nature of competition. They created the following scale to support him and found that it seemed to reduce his anxiety and resulted in decreased competition-based outbursts. In addition to this scale, they wrote individual competition social narratives for bowling, playing games and losing a game to read at school and at home.

(Ned's story was submitted by Susan Leibold and Jackie Novotny, two educators from Turkey Valley Elementary School in Iowa)

off
84

Competition Scale

5	This is not a competition. It is never a game. There are no winners and no losers. This might be personal issues like weight loss or who is the smartest.
4	This is not a game or competition. But someone might get to go first or get to do something that other people don't get to do, like when the teacher tells someone that they can be first in line. This is OK: Take a deep breath.
3	This might be a competition, but some people may not want to compete. This might be like games at recess. Ask other people if they want to have a contest first.
2	This is almost always a competition, but it is usually just for fun. It is important to be a gracious winner and a good loser. Try not to brag if you win, for example, by reminding the losing team that you are the winner. Try not to yell if you lose.
1	This is always a competition, and everyone expects there to be winners and losers. This is like a game between teams in gym class. It is best to be a good winner and a calm loser. Try really hard not to argue if you lose.

When Other People Hear Something Different From What I Thought I Was Saying When I Said That ...

Charles was at a community carnival with his cousin when he observed a third boy "glaring" at his cousin. He decided that this third boy was being a bully and had to be confronted. Although Charles believed his actions were heroic, his words were loud and threatening and his actions appeared aggressive (he pushed the other boy). As a result, Security was called and, according to witnesses, Charles was the culprit.

Needless to say, Charles was not happy; he felt betrayed by an unjust world and had a hard time listening to any alternative perceptions about what happened. Charles' family was also unhappy and confused. His father knew that Charles was a good kid with good intentions, but his words and behavior were sending a different message.

When we first began to process the incident, Charles made a statement that led to a "Powerful Word" Scale. He said, "My dad is afraid I am a vigilante. All I want to be is a protector of innocents." We first reviewed everyone's perspective using cartooning (Gray, 1995). This visual "hard copy" of perspectives was not only our jumping-off point, but also a record of the incident and first meeting.

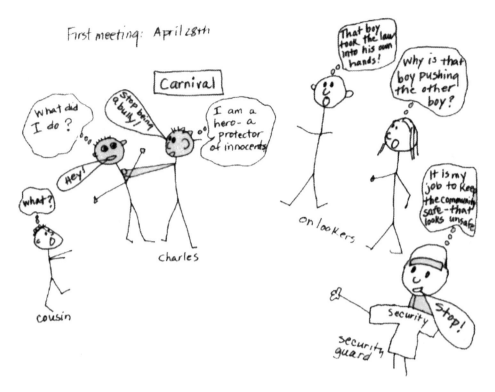

   Charles needed help understanding how his behavior was causing other people to think and how that influenced their actions. Using this scale, Charles was able to visually walk through some differences between how people view a protector vs. a bully. The scale also opened the door to a discussion about the degrees or levels of different behaviors and subsequent punishments. By means of this process, the team was able to identify a few ways Charles might be able to act as a protector without prompting somebody to call Security or him getting in trouble, in general. Charles wanted to be a "protector of innocents," and the team wanted to help him maintain that worthy goal.

   The team generated a list of people who might be identified as protectors. Charles and his teacher agreed that everybody on the list was a protector. They discussed the personal and behavioral traits one might see in a protector, generated some ideas about the words a protector might use, and compared real-life protectors to super heroes, avatars, and characters from TV shows. It was helpful to have Charles think about which super hero behaviors might be good in the real world and which ones would be illegal.

Target Word(s): Vigilante, Protector of Innocents	The Power of Meaning Word Scale
Rating	Word and Meaning
5	**Monster** This is a very cruel person who doesn't think about the well-being of others at all. This type of person hurts other people and is very, very scary!
4	**Vigilante** These are people who take the law into their own hands and punish people like bullies. They might mean well, but they are breaking the law.
3	**Professional Peacekeeper** Military, police, Transportation Security Administration (TSA), crossing guard, etc.
2	**Protector** Moms and dads; older brothers and sisters; babysitters. If you are bigger and stronger – defender of younger, helpless.
1	**Helper** Volunteers at food pantry; people who read to little kids; people who shovel the sidewalk for their older neighbors.

The Ultimate Goal

When a person becomes familiar with a strategy and begins to use it across environments, situations, and people, that is called generalization. And that is pretty exciting. Since self-management and self-awareness are two of the primary goals of using the 5-Point Scale, the following three scales are reason for great celebration! These scales were developed by the students themselves after they had been introduced to the 5-Point Scale.

The first scale was developed by Harrison Scott, a 10-year-old boy from Vancouver, BC, Canada, who loves *Star Wars*. After using a 5-Point Scale to understand issues of emotional self-regulation, Harrison announced to his mother, Leah, that he would like to create a scale using the different planets in *Star Wars*. He came up with the title *Search Your Feelings*, a clever reference to a line by Darth Vader to Luke Skywalker that symbolizes one of the most emotional scenes in the movie. It is amazing that Harrison not only related his scale to this very emotional moment in the movie, but also knew all of the planets and was able to assign them feelings based on their characteristics.

Search Your Feelings Star Wars Feelings Chart	
Original Idea: Harrison Scott · · · · · Created by Harrison Scott and Leah Kelley	
Mustafar: A hot feeling, full of anger and revenge – losing control ... a volcano planet	
Geonosis: Full of too much energy ... getting mad and not making positive decisions	
Tantooine: A very rough feeling – it is uncomfortable ... it is a desert planet	
Hoth: A sad and cold feeling ... deep breaths, a hug, or talking can bring calm	
Dantooine: A peaceful place known to the Republic ... a calm feeling	

The second scale was developed by Eleanor Quayle, a third grader who was studying scales to learn about emotions and feelings. Eleanor's teacher gave her a worksheet from the original 5-Point Scale book (page 71) and asked her to draw pictures of herself at different levels of anxiety – from a level of no anxiety to being out of control. The teacher then asked Eleanor to fill in the blanks describing what each level feels like and what she can *try to do* when she feels that way. Finally, the teacher took pictures of Eleanor demonstrating how she might look at each level and asked Eleanor to find where they belong on the scale.

Name: Eleanor   My five point   Scale

Rating	Looks like	Feels like	I can *try* to
	Whoa! yay! John Hooray	very angry/mad feeling evil / being hyper having too much fun	make things better / be calm
	time	Upset/feeling like complaining My Tummy hurts! I'm hungry / feeling mischievous	take a time out!! / take deep breaths! be calm.
		happy enjoying life / not bored	keep concetrating/ paying attention / keep busy
		feeling a little drowsy / sleepy/feeling good	rest for a little while / take a break
		falling asleep / dozing off	stretching / do something you like at school

The Incredible 5-Point Scale

Tatum Anderson, an elementary school student who had learned how to rate her problems using the scale, developed the third scale. One day, Tatum was in gym class and two students began to argue over the rules of a game. The argument escalated to the point of becoming physical.

Tatum recognized that some training was needed to help the students understand that their reaction to the problem was disproportionate to the problem itself. That is when she independently added the Reaction Scale portion of her scale.

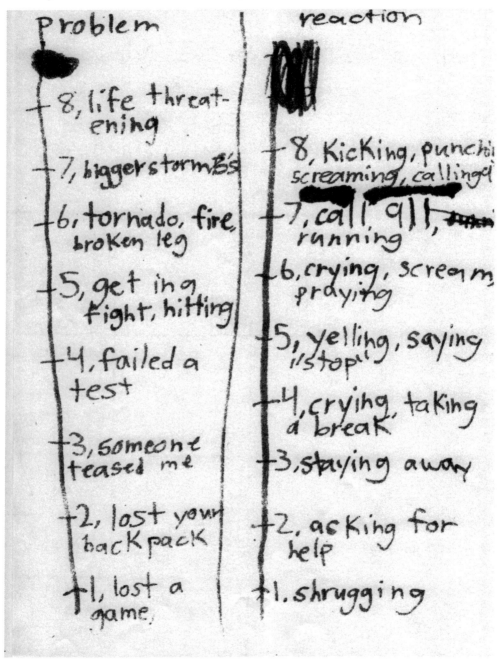

(Thank you to the wonderfully gracious and supportive families, Leah Kelley, Amy and Scott Anderson and Luann and Peter Quayle, for sharing their children's work; thanks also goes to Joyce Santo, a teacher from Roseville, Minnesota, for her help with this section)

Sample Goals and Objectives Related to the Use of the 5-Point Scale

One of the questions we get often is, "How do you write goals and objectives for using the 5-Point Scale?" We asked some of the teachers we know to give us examples of how they have included use of the scale in their students' individualized education programs (IEP). We hope you find these examples helpful in your own planning.

Andrew

Goal:

By May 2013, Andrew will improve his self-monitoring skills related to his voice volume by referring to his Voice Volume Scale when directed by an adult and adjusting his volume, whether up or down, from a level of 0% follow-through to a level of 70% follow-through **during a 2-week charting period.**

Objectives:

Given direct teaching and modeling, Andrew will identify his levels of voice volume on the Voice Volume Scale with 70% accuracy, as measured by clinician data over 8 consecutive data days.

Given direct teaching and modeling, Andrew will change the volume of his voice when an adult points to a designated volume level on his Voice Volume Scale in 7/10 opportunities, as measured by clinician data **over 8 consecutive data days.**

Sally

Goal:

When frustrated, Sally will determine the size of the problem using the 5-Point Problem Scale, describe her emotional reaction to the problem based on the size, minimize her emotional response to the problem, and decrease the amount of time it takes her to recover from the problem in 70% of the **problem** situations over 20 consecutive data days.

Objectives:

Given a situation that involves a "3" problem that is moderately frustrating, Sally will accurately determine the size of the problem using 5-Point Scale language, in 3 out of 4 opportunities, as measured by teacher data over 10 consecutive data days.

The Incredible 5-Point Scale

Given a "4" level problem as defined on her 5-Point Problem Scale, Sally will state the problem and use a predetermined strategy to decrease her emotional response in 4 out of 5 opportunities, as measured by teacher data taken over 10 consecutive data days.

Sven

Goal:

Sven will improve his ability to self-monitor and regulate his emotions by utilizing a 5-Point Stress Scale and accessing self-calming strategies, including his personal journal, the calming area, Theraputty, a labyrinth, or music/headphones, from a level of not monitoring or regulating his emotions to a level of doing so with a nonverbal staff prompt 75% of the time over 10 consecutive data days.

Objective:

Given the opportunity to self-monitor his emotions through the use of a 5-Point Stress Scale and access to calming strategies, Sven will monitor and regulate his emotions 90% of the time over a period of 8 data-taking days with 3 nonverbal staff prompts, as measured by teacher, by January 2012. With 1 nonverbal staff prompt by June of 2012.

Goal:

Sven will utilize an individualized 5-Point Stress Scale worksheet to identify things that cause him stress, what it looks like, and what it feels like. He will identify strategies he can use to prevent stress and activities to control emotions with 70% accuracy over 30 days of data taking.

Objective:

Given an individualized 5-Point Stress Scale worksheet and matching data sheet, Sven will check in with his teacher 3 times a day to practice rating his stress level, as noted on his data sheet, throughout the second grading term.

Given a thrice-daily check-in on his 5-Point Stress Scale and worksheet, Sven will choose and carry out a calming strategy that corresponds to his rating, throughout the third grading term, as noted by teacher data.

Steve

Goal:

Steve will increase his ability to accurately communicate how he feels when he is frustrated, from a level of yelling, crying, stomping his feet, and/or throwing materials to a level of identifying how his body feels and participating in calming techniques over 30 data days.

Objectives:

Given a situation that makes Steve feel frustrated and a 5-Point Scale visual support, Steve will verbally state what number his body is at before participating in negative behavior (yelling, crying, stomping his feet, and/or throwing materials). He can currently complete this skill for 20% of the opportunities provided and is expected to complete this skill for 70% of the opportunities provided over 10 consecutive data days, as measured by the special education staff, by his next annual IEP.

Given a situation that makes Steve feel frustrated and a 5-Point Scale visual support on which Steve is already able to identify the number where his body is, Steve will participate in a calming technique identified on his 5-Point Scale. He can currently complete this skill in 10% of the opportunities provided and will be expected to complete this skill 70% of the opportunities provided over 10 consecutive data days, as measured by the special education staff, by his next annual IEP.

Larry

Goal:

Larry will increase his ability to cope when he is denied a preferred activity, from a level of participating in negative behaviors (running, hitting, spitting, throwing, attempting to bite) to a level of stating how he feels and participating in calming techniques by the end of the term, as recorded over 15 data days.

Objectives:

Given a 5-Point Mad Scale and a visual scenario of what might make him mad, Larry will state how the situation would make him feel and participate in a calming technique. Larry currently completes this skill on 30% of the opportunities provided. He is expected to complete this skill on 60% of the opportunities provided by his Progress Report 1, as measured by the special education staff; on 80% by Progress Report 2, again measured through teacher data.

Joe

Goal:

Joe will increase his ability to maintain calm, focused attention on school activities from a level of doing so during tasks, environments, and people that are familiar to a level of being able to tolerate change in tasks, environment, and people given prior warning and a 5-Point Anxiety Scale.

The Plan:

- Joe will accurately identify his anxiety level on a 5-Point Scale 5 times daily.
- Joe will identify the reason for any increased anxiety 3/5 occurrences over 10 consecutive data days.
- Joe will develop a "toolbox" of five strategies he can use to calm himself when he rates himself at a 3 or above.
- Joe will correctly identify events and situations that cause him anxiety using the activity *A 5 Could Make Me Lose Control!* (Buron, 2007).
- Joe will connect his toolbox strategies to stressful situations and co-create a plan for using these strategies when the situations occur naturally.

The Incredible 5-Point Scale

Objectives:
Given a mildly challenging situation, Joe will choose and use a strategy from his toolbox, 4/5 times per day over 3 sessions.

Given a mildly challenging situation, Joe will generate three possible options for a course of action 4/5 times over 3 sessions.

Given a social situation, Joe will accurately predict the outcomes for a given course of action with 70% accuracy, as recorded by teacher data over 15 consecutive data days.

More Objectives

Jeff
Given staff prompting and his visual scale, Jeff will identify where his anxiety is (or was, if processing after an incident) and problem-solve the situation on 4 out of 5 occasions, as measured by classroom staff over 10 consecutive data days.

Sven
Given instruction in the use of the Positive Interaction Scale, Sven will work with staff to come up with a list of 5-7 interaction skills he can use in situations with peers and staff to gain a positive outcome in 3/5 trials, as measured by a staff data sheet over 10 consecutive data days.

Tom
Given practice using his 5-Point Scale as a prompt, Tom will independently choose and use 3 calming strategies (visual, nonverbal, breaks, hands-on, etc.) to manage his anxiety in 3 out of 5 opportunities, as measured by classroom staff over 10 consecutive data days.

Given a 5-Point Voice Scale, Tom will positively respond to a prearranged nonverbal signal to support him in modifying his tone and/or volume of voice, as recorded by his teacher on 10 consecutive data days.

Mark
Given a 5-Point Anxiety Scale and a social scenario, Mark will correctly identify another person's level of emotional response, as measured by daily staff documentation on 15 consecutive data days, by December 2012.

Jeremy
Given a 5-Point Anxiety Scale, Jeremy will recognize the level where he is and use the prescribed strategies to maintain a calm and organized state 95% of the time, as recorded in daily behavior data over 15 consecutive data days.

Andy

Given a 5-Point Scale "check-in" system and plan, Andy will rate the level of his anxiety 3 times daily and record his rating on a weekly chart over 30 consecutive data days.

Given a 5-Point Scale "check-in" system and plan, Andy will respond to his ratings 3 times daily by engaging in predetermined calming activities, as observed and recorded by his teacher on 30 consecutive data days.

(Our thanks to the following educators for their contributions to this section:
Donna Asher, a teacher from Minneapolis, Minnesota
Janet McDonald, a teacher from Minneapolis, Minnesota
Kelly Norden, a teacher from Minneapolis, Minnesota
Adrienne Jonas, a teacher from Minneapolis, Minnesota
Holly Paschke, a Speech Pathologist from Clover Ridge Elementary School, Minnesota
Joyce Santo, a teacher from Roseville, Minnesota)

References

Asperger, H. (1944). Die 'Autistichen Psychopathen' im Kindersalter. *Archiv für Psychiatrie und Nervenkrankheiten, 117,* 76-136.

Aspy, R., & Grossman, B. (2011). *The Ziggurat model: A framework for designing comprehensive interventions for high-functioning individuals with autism spectrum disorders, release 2.0.* Shawnee Mission, KS: AAPC Publishing.

Buron, K. D. (2006). *When my worries get too big!* Shawnee Mission, KS: AAPC Publishing.

Buron, K. D. (2007). *A 5 could make me lose control!* Shawnee Mission, KS: AAPC Publishing.

Buron, K. D., & Curtis, M. (2009). *The 5-point scale and anxiety curve poster.* Shawnee Mission, KS: AAPC Publishing.

Castorina, L. L., & Negri, L. M. (2011). The inclusion of sibling in social skills training groups for boys with Asperger Syndrome. *Journal of Autism and Developmental Disorders, 41,* 73-81.

Gagnon, E. (2001). *Power cards.* Shawnee Mission, KS: AAPC Publishing.

Golan, O., & Baron-Cohen, S. (2008). Systemizing emotions: Using interactive multimedia as a teaching tool. In K. D. Buron & P. Wolfberg (Eds.), *Learners on the autism spectrum: Preparing highly qualified educators* (pp. 234-253). Shawnee Mission, KS: AAPC Publishing.

Goleman, D. (2011). *The brain and emotional intelligence: New insights.* Northhampton, MA: More Than Sounds LLC.

Gray, C. (1995). *Social stories unlimited: Social stories and comic strip conversations.* Jenison, MI: Jenison Public Schools.

Kanner, L. (1943). Autistic disturbances of affective contact. *Nervous Child, 2,* 227-250.

Sansosti, F. (2010). Teaching social skills to children with autism spectrum disorders using tiers of support: A guide for school-based professionals. *Psychology in the Schools, 47*(3), 257-281.

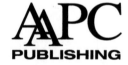

P.O. Box 23173
Shawnee Mission, Kansas 66283-0173
www.aapcpublishing.net